AN INTRODUCTION TO
MACROBIOTICS

A refreshingly new, clear and optimistic view of the physical, mental
and emotional benefits of a macrobiotic lifestyle.

AN INTRODUCTION TO
MACROBIOTICS

The Natural Way to Health and Happiness

by

Oliver Cowmeadow

THORSONS PUBLISHING GROUP
Wellingborough, Northamptonshire

First published 1987

© OLIVER COWMEADOW 1987

British Library Cataloguing in Publication Data

Cowmeadow, Oliver
An introduction to macrobiotics: the
natural way to health and happiness.
1. Macrobiotic diet
I. Title
613.2'6   RM235

ISBN 0-7225-1414-X

*Published by Thorsons Publishers Limited,
Wellingborough, Northamptonshire, NN8 2RQ, England*

Printed in Great Britain by The Guernsey Press, Vale, Guernsey

3 5 7 9 10 8 6 4 2

CONTENTS

ACKNOWLEDGEMENTS

I would like to give my deep thanks to all my teachers for their help and inspiration in opening my eyes to the possibilities of life, especially to Michio and Aveline Kushi, Denny and Judy Waxman, Rik Vermuyten, Bill Tara, Adelbert and Wieke Nelissen, and Ferro Ledvinka. Also to Niel Gulliver, Peter and Montse Bradford, Jon Sandifer, and many friends for sharing their ideas and experiences that have contributed to this book. And to Michele, my wife and companion, without whose help and encouragement this book would probably not have been written, and to my daughter Isolde who has taught me the wonder of life. I hope that through the help of these people I may pass on to readers a way to realize the endless adventure of life.

INTRODUCTION

The quality of our health and lives depends on what we think is possible for us. This book will greatly expand the horizons of what you thought was possible, enhancing and nourishing all aspects of your well-being. It offers a totally new way of understanding your life, and the practical means for creating vitality and health, a positive and happy emotional and mental experience, harmonious and rewarding relationships, and an increased awareness of life.

In our modern society the most basic aspects of life have been forgotten—how to eat, how to be healthy, how to be happy. Hundreds of books have been written on how to eat healthily, how to enjoy sex, how to reduce stress and how to find happiness. The human being is the only animal on earth who has forgotten these basics of living! A crocodile, a sparrow, an elephant all know what to eat and how to behave. How have we forgotten what all other creatures instinctively know?

Macrobiotics offers a way for us to recover our intuition, our common-sense knowledge of what to eat and how to act to create health and happiness. The word macrobiotics is made up of the Greek words *macro* meaning large, and *bios* meaning life, so macrobiotics means *large-life*, or looking at life from the broadest possible view. With this broad view we can see that there is a definite order in all that happens in nature and the universe. Everywhere one looks the same patterns of rhythmic change can be found. As we are one small part of nature, our lives also follow the same patterns of change or natural laws.

These natural laws were once known by many ancient cultures around the world, including the American Indians, Aztecs and Incas, Celts, ancient Egyptians and Greeks, and peoples in the Middle East, India and the Far East. They have largely been forgotten in the modern world. Fortunately, an understanding of these laws has remained intact until recent times in China, Japan and other parts of the Far East. It is from these ancient sources of wisdom that macrobiotics has drawn its unique view of life, and brought it up to date for life in our modern world.

By studying these natural laws we can recover our understanding of how to create health and happiness in our lives. We can turn sickness into health, unhappiness into happiness, conflict into harmony, creating our lives as we want rather than being at the mercy of our circumstances. As a fundamental way of recreating our health this book gives a diet plan and ways of cooking these foods. However, this is not just another diet to be blindly or rigidly followed, but some guidelines from which you can develop your own understanding of how to eat to optimize your health and psychological well-being. If you spend some time following these guidelines, you will discover through your own experiences the truth of the macrobiotic principles of healthy eating. After a while, choosing a balanced and healthy diet becomes part of your own common-sense approach to life.

This book begins by giving a new view of health and life from the macrobiotic point of view. It then goes on to the theory of how we can increase our health and happiness. Finally, the chapters with menu plans and recipes give you the practical means for beginning on the improvement of your diet and health. Altogether these chapters give you the vision, understanding, and practical means to begin on a new path to a fuller and more rewarding life. At first some of the ideas may seem strange or foreign, but keep reading and experimenting with them, and with each passing day you will discover more of their basic truth. Explore this new approach to life to the full, because the rewards for your efforts could be far greater than you ever expected.

The appendix at the end of the book gives information to help you continue your study and practice of macrobiotics, with a list of further books to read, addresses for finding out about classes and other help, and mail-order shops selling typical foods for the macrobiotic way of eating in case you have any difficulty in finding them. There are many exciting aspects of the macrobiotic understanding that cannot be covered in this book, but which you are encouraged to find out about. This includes the study of physiognomy and body language as a way of reading our constitutional strengths and potentials and present state of health;

Do-in exercises for strengthening and harmonizing our energy flow for physical health and spiritual growth; oriental astrology for understanding our individual destiny and that of humanity as a whole; and shiatus as a way of natural self-health care.

CHAPTER ONE

THE HISTORY
OF MACROBIOTICS

A brief look at the origin and history of macrobiotics is useful in understanding its approach to health, and putting this into context with our modern Western way of life. The person who first used the word 'macrobiotics' in this context was George Ohsawa, who was born in Kyoto in Japan in 1893. At the age of 18, he developed tuberculosis of the lungs and intestines, and was told by doctors of Western medicine that he had only a few months to live. However, he chanced upon a book applying ancient oriental medicine to food and health. He tried the recommended diet, based on whole brown rice, soup and vegetables, and completely cured himself.

Later, Ohsawa went on to study in greater depth the application of oriental philosophy to diet, health, and physiognomy (the art of reading features in the face that reveal a person's character and state of health) and helped many hundreds of people recover from sickness through his advice on diet and lifestyle. He went on to investigate the broader aspects of Far Eastern philosophy, and distilled its essence in a form more easily understood by the modern mind, which he called macrobiotics.

The wide-scale introduction of macrobiotics in the West began in 1953, when Ohsawa travelled with his wife, Lima, to Europe and America. From this time up until his death in 1966 he was very active teaching and writing, and introduced many thousands of people to the macrobiotic understanding of life.

After his death, many of Ohsawa's friends and students continued to teach the macrobiotic philosophy and its practical application to daily life. Foremost among them is Michio Kushi and his wife Aveline. When they first met Ohsawa in Japan after the Second World War, Michio Kushi's main interest was in how to create world peace. Ohsawa introduced him to the idea of applying oriental philosophy and its dietary principles to establishing peace, through the transformation of individuals to health and happiness. The Kushis moved to America, and have been teaching macrobiotic ideas ever since. They now live in Boston, and regularly travel to many parts of the world, teaching and giving individual help to thousands of people. Through the vision and tireless efforts of Kushi and other teachers, centres of macrobiotic teaching have been set up across North America, in Britain and most other European countries, and in almost every continent of the world. These offer a wide range of classes on macrobiotic philosophy and its practical application to a healthier way of living and eating. A list of these centres can be obtained from the addresses given on page 158.

Interest in macrobiotics was instrumental in beginning the natural foods revolution, with a return to whole and unchemicalized foods. Now many of the foods first introduced by people following macrobiotic guidelines are widely available in health and wholefood shops, including brown rice and other whole grains, soya beans and their products like tofu, shoyu soy sauce and miso, sea vegetables, rice cakes and many others.

The history of macrobiotics can be traced from the ancient traditions of China and the Far East, through George Ohsawa who brought these ideas to the West, to Michio Kushi and others who have spread its understanding across the Western world. It is still based on the essence of the oriental understanding of life, using the concepts of yin and yang; these two symbols remain because there are no words in the English language with the same meaning. Ohsawa presented these ancient truths in a new and dynamic form, and with Kushi these ideas have been integrated with the Western view of the world, including science, medicine, psychology and philosophy.

With the spread of macrobiotics to many different countries, the diet is becoming adapted to the traditional foods of different regions. It no longer appears particularly Japanese, and is not just a brown rice diet! It is the macrobiotic principles of how to eat a balanced and healthy diet that are universal, and not the specific foods included in the diet. In fact, the traditional diets of people around the world are very similar in their basic plan, with whole cereal grains or bread made from them forming the largest part, and *local* vegetables, beans and pulses, and sometimes small quantities of fish or meat making up the rest of the diet. Macrobiotic guidelines on healthier eating follow this same basic plan, and so bring us back to our own traditional way of eating.

These changes are making the macrobiotic philosophy and diet more appealing and easily understood by people in Western countries seeking a healthier way of life. Although putting these into practice requires study and seemingly big adjustments in diet and lifestyle, more and more people are discovering the underlying truth of this way of life, and the great benefits of putting its principles into practice in their daily lives.

CHAPTER TWO

A NEW VIEW OF HEALTH

Health is the foundation of our life. With it, we can enjoy all the varied experiences that life offers us; without it, our lives become limited by sickness and difficulties.

Everybody wants health, yet somehow it is rare to find a person one could call really whole and healthy. Most people do not realize the extent to which they could enjoy far greater health.

The most common idea of health is a negative one—to have no obvious sickness or signs of ill-health. This is perhaps not surprising as sickness is so common in modern society that to be free of it for a time seems like a great gift. However, we should be able to expect far more in health terms than just avoiding sickness. A more positive idea of health is *enjoying an open and positive emotional life with harmonious and rewarding relations with other people and nature, having the vitality and gratitude to enjoy everything one does, and the clarity and freedom to create one's life as one chooses.*

In finding health, the first stage is therefore learning how to prevent ourselves from becoming sick. We can then learn how to increase the positive aspects of health, which makes way for the free choice of the many things that we want to do in life. Unfortunately, the modern understanding of health fails at the first hurdle—the way to prevent sickness. Presently we are faced with an epidemic of serious health problems affecting nearly every individual and family at some time. In Britain, nearly half of all deaths today are due to heart disease, strokes, and other disorders of the circulatory system. Just under a quarter of people die from cancer, and it is estimated that one in three people will suffer from this disease at sometime during their lifetime. One in a hundred people have been diagnosed as having diabetes, and another one in a hundred probably have undiagnosed diabetes. Two million people suffer from asthma, including one in twenty schoolchildren. Migraine headaches are estimated to affect six million people, and epilepsy 300,000. To add to the problem, new diseases such as AIDS are appearing. Various emotional and mental problems are on the increase, with a large proportion of the population taking tranquillizers, anti-depressants, and other mind-altering drugs.

In the face of this problem, tremendous amounts of time, money and effort are being spent to find answers and cures. Yet diabetes, many forms of cancer, AIDS, other forms of degenerative disease, and mental illness are still very much on the increase. These researches have not come up with the answer to the question of what causes these diseases, or even many common ailments like headaches, skin ailments or back pain.

The failure of the modern understanding of health lies in its underlying way of thinking and view of life. The macrobiotic understanding of life offers a refreshingly new view, with which we can not only prevent serious sickness, but also maximize the positive aspects of health and our overall quality of life.

A WIDER VIEW OF HEALTH

Currently, the main way of trying to understand life and health is to divide the world into small parts, and to study these parts in greater and greater detail. This *microscopic* way of thinking has created a wealth of knowledge about the detailed working of atoms, stars, cells, plants, animals and other parts of nature, but misses the *big picture* of how all these details are related to each other and work together as a whole. Our modern knowledge is made up of fragments, rather like the pieces of a jig-saw puzzle, without knowing how they can all be fitted together.

In the field of health, this approach has created blood specialists, bone specialists, eye specialists, psychiatrists, psychologists, nutritionalists, and a host of other -ists. While this detailed understanding can be very useful, it does not take into account how all these individual aspects fit together to form a whole person with his or her food, activities, natural environment, emotions and social relations, and other influences on his health.

The macrobiotic approach to health takes the broadest view possible, with a *macroscopic* way of looking at ourselves and nature. This provides the *whole picture* so that the pieces of the jig-saw puzzle can be easily fitted together. In the big view, we can see that we are not isolated units, but are intimately connected with our environment. We are completely dependent on the sun, air, water, and soil of our natural environment to continually nurture us. We take these four elements into ourselves in the concentrated form of food grown in the soil. Plants transform them into the nutrients we need to live. We also take in vibrations such as sounds, ideas and other forms of communication between people. These different kinds of energy and matter are transformed, and then given out as faeces, urine and perspiration, carbon dioxide, in our activities and behaviour, and as our emotional expression and communication. This wholistic view of ourselves is illustrated in figure I.

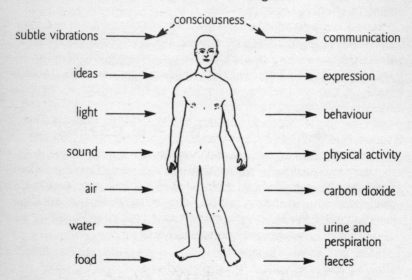

consciousness

subtle vibrations ——→   ——→ communication

ideas ——→   ——→ expression

light ——→   ——→ behaviour

sound ——→   ——→ physical activity

air ——→   ——→ carbon dioxide

water ——→   ——→ urine and perspiration

food ——→   ——→ faeces

Figure I. *A macroscopic view of ourselves in our environment.*

In this broader macroscopic view, our internal health depends on what we take in from our environment, and what we give back out. We have little control over some of these, such as the quality of light or air we take in, but have great control over others. We can choose the ideas we receive, think about and apply in our lives (like choosing to read this book!) We can improve the efficiency of our breathing and increase the amount of oxygen and energy that we get from the air. Everyone can make changes to a healthier way of eating. We can increase our level of physical activity, either within our daily routine or with yoga, sports, martial arts and other exercise programmes. With thought, we can change the way we behave and express ourselves, and how we communicate and relate with other people.

Of all these influences on our health, food is perhaps the greatest. Every day we eat, and from this food we daily recreate our blood and our cells: the whole body is made from food transformed into living tissues. Just tap your chest—what you feel is the food you ate yesterday, and the day before that, and the day before that! We also have almost complete control over what we eat, so through our choice of food we can have enormous control over our health.

It is with our consciousness that we choose what we take in and give out, so the key to increasing our health is raising our consciousness of which foods, activities, and ways of relating to other people and to nature lead to greater health. The macrobiotic understanding of the order in nature gives us great insight into how we can do this. A basic principle is creating a balance in what we take in and what we give out, by which we can prevent serious sickness and optimize our physical health, create a positive emotional life, and a balance in our moods and perspectives on life.

The rest of this book will explain in more detail how you can achieve this balance. Before we look at that, however, we can consider the advantages of this understanding for our physical health, choice of diet, and emotional and mental health. To make these new views clearer, the key differences between the common modern approach to health and the macrobiotic approach are summarized in figure 2.

A NEW VIEW OF PHYSICAL HEALTH

The old saying prevention is better than cure has great truth. Unfortunately, the modern understanding of health has focused on *sickness* and sick people, and on how to deal with sickness once it has occurred. Macrobiotics has the opposite focus, on *health* and healthy people, and how we can prevent ourselves becoming sick and optimize our overall health. It allows us to become self-reliant in our everyday health care.

Modern medicine has an important role in modern life, especially in the treatment of accidents and emergencies. However, we can largely avoid

	Modern Approach	Macrobiotic Approach
view of life	microscopic	macroscopic
understanding	fragmentary	wholistic
responsibility for health care	in hands of experts	in own hands
focus	on disease and its cure	on prevention and maximizing health
approach to sickness	symptomatic	changing causes
method of treatment	artificial	natural
side-effects of treatment	great	little or none
view of the world	dualistic	harmony between opposites
attitude to nature	an enemy to be fought	a friend to live in harmony with
attitude to sickness	an unnatural intrusion	a natural result of past lifestyle
response to sickness	blame external factors	self-reflection and self-change

Figure 2. *Key differences between the modern and macrobiotic approaches to health and sickness.*

having to resort to it for the treatment of common sicknesses. The extent to which we can do this is shown by the experience of thousands of people currently practising the macrobiotic way to health, and who have continued to seriously study and apply the macrobiotic approach to health care—none has developed cancer, diabetes, multiple sclerosis, or many other degenerative diseases. Many have experienced a new calmness and ease, with a reduction in tension and stress, and a far more positive and happy outlook on life.

The beauty of the macrobiotic approach to health is that it uses terms that anyone can understand. It has a simple understanding of how nature and people work; it deals with foods, emotions and attitudes in everyday language; and everyone can develop a sense of balance in their health and lives. Instead of feeling totally ignorant about the workings of our body, we can all learn the basics of self-health care.

As we live in a world where disease is very common, we can also look at the benefits of the macrobiotic approach to sickness. You may be suffering from a health problem yourself, or know other people who are. Apart from the more serious degenerative illnesses, there are many less serious problems that limit one's enjoyment of life, including frequent colds, coughs and infections, pre-mentrual tension, painful periods, earache and partial deafness, headaches and migraines, hayfever, poor sleep, and a general lack of vitality. All of these can be improved by adopting the macrobiotic way of life.

A great advantage of the macrobiotic approach is that it helps us to understand *the fundamental causes of illness*, which lie in the way we have chosen what to take in from and give back to our environment. By changing to a more balanced way of eating and other more healthy ways of living, we can usually avoid having to use various symptomatic treatments like drugs and medications. Many people feel a great relief when they understand the cause of their problem, and the knowledge that they can do something about it themselves can inspire them to make changes to a healthier way of living.

One benefit of looking at the causes of a health problem and changing to a healthier way of living is that one can avoid the harmful side-effects of most symptomatic treatments. Modern symptomatic treatments are becoming increasingly artificial, including drugs, surgery, and radiation. Any artificial treatment has damaging effects on a person's overall health, and the more unnatural or artificial it is, the greater the harm. By making changes in one's daily eating and lifestyle, health is restored using the body's own natural healing powers and those of food, air, sun and appropriate activities. While modern artificial treatments are sometimes essential to save life, in most cases of sickness more natural methods can successfully restore health.

With the macrobiotic way to health, we can develop a deep harmony in our thinking and lives without conflict and antagonism. Most people agree that we should be taking care of our natural environment and of other people in the world, living in harmony with them. However, an exception is often made when it comes to illness—the bacteria, virus or other natural force causing the illness is seen as an *unnatural intrusion* into the body, to be fought and conquered. This *dualistic* way of seeing the world divides life into two opposite categories that are antagonistic or at war with each other. The macrobiotic view of the world recognizes these opposite categories, and uses yin and yang to understand them, but sees that they are *complementary*, each helping the other. Nature is our friend, it has created us, continues to nurture us, and provides all that we need to enjoy good health. This includes bacteria, viruses and all other natural forces. The naturally occuring micro-organisms in the soil break down organic matter to provide food for the plants that we eat, and similarly those in our intestines aid our digestion of food and produce various vitamins that we absorb. We could not live without these friendly and helpful creatures.

If we accept this harmony, we can take a very different attitude in approaching health problems. If we become sick, we cannot blame these external micro-organisms or forces, which are our friends. Instead, we must realize that it is we who have caused our problems, because we have not understood how to eat, think and act in harmony with nature's laws. If we harbour harmful bacteria and viruses, it is because we have created a poor blood and body quality that has allowed these organisms to enter and thrive. Sickness is a *natural result* of our past way of thinking and behaving. If we are humble in the face of nature, and prepared to learn from her and change our ways, then we can restore our health. Through our own self-reflection, self-examination and self-change we can free ourselves of sickness and enjoy health and happiness for the rest of our lives.

A few examples of these two approaches to some specific health problems will make the advantages of the macrobiotic approach clearer. The first is cancer, probably the most feared disease in modern society. In the last few decades there has been an enormous effort to find its cure, with over a billion pounds spent every year on research, yet still we do not have the answer. This research primarily focusses on the cancerous cells, molecules within them, carcinogenic chemicals, and the possible role of viruses in causing cancer. It mainly considers how to treat the symptoms of cancer—that is, how to remove or kill off the cancerous cells once they have arisen in the body. This has yielded increasingly artificial treatments, including surgery, the use of radiation, and of very powerful drugs which do much harm to the whole body by killing off many healthy cells. Because of the highly technical forms of treatment, the cancer patient often feels totally out of control of the situation. The attitude towards the cancer is that it is an unnatural intrusion into the body, an enemy to be fought at all costs. Little if any consideration is given to how the patient may help himself through changes in diet, attitude and lifestyle.

With our broader view, the causes of cancer can be understood in the same way as any other disease. Cancer is the natural result of unhealthy daily eating, activities, and behaviour over many years. With this understanding, it is quite possible for us to prevent cancer ever occurring. If it does occur, however, the broad view recognizes that using natural means can greatly aid recovery by strengthening the individual rather than by attacking the cancer; by giving life rather than by killing. This is based on regarding the cancer as a friend, a welcome call from nature telling us that we have strayed in our understanding and ways, and stimulating change to a healthier and more rewarding way of living.

A second example is the rise of infertility in modern society. A recent medical report stated that there are probably nearly 300,000 childless couples between the ages of 24 and 35 in Britain, for whom 'test tube' fertilization is the only hope for having a family. This approach is obviously highly symptomatic and artificial, and possibly has enormous side-effects. While this technique seems to produce physically normal babies, the psychological and spiritual effects on people who began their life in a test tube rather than their mother's womb is largely unknown. There is much evidence that a mother and her child have a very intimate relationship during pregnancy, which has a great effect on the child's future emotional and mental life. The events surrounding the beginning of life most probably have an even greater effect.

The macrobiotic approach offers a more natural solution to this problem, which is safer for the parents, offspring, and future generations to come. Being unable to conceive offers a stimulus for deep self-reflection by a couple, to find the cause of their infertility and make changes in their diet and lifestyle to restore their health and capacity to bring forth new life. This can bring about greater health and happiness for the parents themselves, and also greater reward for them in raising their children in good health and with the greatest chance of living a full and interesting life.

A third example is the new disease presently sweeping through the world—AIDS, or auto-immune deficiency syndrome. A particularly noticeable feature is the deep and widespread fear it has produced because people do not understand its cause, or know whether they may be susceptible to developing it, and how they can prevent themselves from suffering from it. With an understanding of macrobiotic principles, this fear is completely dissolved. In general terms, the cause of AIDS is the same as any other disease, an unnatural way of living and eating. This causes a degeneration in health that makes the body susceptible to viruses in general, including the AIDS virus. By changing to a healthier way of eating and living using macrobiotic principles, we can improve our health so that we are no longer a suitable home for this disease. Early studies in New York using the macrobiotic approach to curing AIDS are also producing promising results, which are better than anything else yet tried. This disease shows the possibilities of the macrobiotic approach for increasing our quality of life—with it, we can rid ourselves of the fear of serious illness, making way for a full and long life of health and happiness.

A NEW VIEW OF FOOD AND DIET

There are now many ideas on what constitutes a healthy diet, but these often contradict each other and present a very confusing picture. This is because most of the current ideas on healthy eating look at only one aspect of health and do not take in the whole picture. For example, the modern scientific approach analyses food into its nutritional components like carbohydrate, protein, fat, minerals, vitamins and fibre, to ensure that we get enough of these different nutrients. We can avoid suffering from nutritional deficiences in this way but it does not ensure overall health. Many people who get all the recommended amounts of nutrients still become ill.

Other popular diets include eating high-fibre foods to improve digestion, eating different food groups only in certain combinations for easier digestion, eating plenty of fruit to obtain adequate vitamin C, and eating primarily raw foods to optimize the life force of food. All these approaches are limited to one particular aspect of health so, although they may be valuable in their own way, they do not ensure overall health.

The macrobiotic understanding of food and diet has several advantages:

1. It cuts through confusion with a comprehensive way of understanding the effects of different foods and diets. This is based on an understanding

of the unique energetic quality of different foods using yin and yang. In this way we can understand the effects of every food on specific organs and bodily functions, on our moods and emotions, and on our perceptions and thinking. This enables us to design a diet to optimize our overall health and quality of life.

2. Many diets involve the counting of calories and different nutrients. This is based on the chemical analysis of foods, which is beyond our normal perception. The macrobiotic approach talks of food as we know it: as bread, sugar, meat, vegetables and so on, so that everyone can develop an intuitive understanding of the quality and effects of different foods, and choose their own diet appropriately.

3. The macrobiotic approach to healthy eating is flexible and can be adapted to every person's individual needs. Most other diets make across-the-board recommendations for everyone, but common sense tells us that we each need to eat differently for our health. Macrobiotic principles give a simple understanding of how we can adapt our food to suit these differing needs, according to differences in climate, season, age, activity, and so on.

A NEW VIEW OF EMOTIONAL AND MENTAL HEALTH

Emotional and mental health is commonly viewed in the same way as physical health—with a microscopic way of thinking, concentrating on the problems and ignoring the larger view of the whole person and his or her relationship with their environment. Problems are often labelled according to their symptoms, and treatments focus on changing these symptoms rather than the whole person. The most common treatment is to use drugs like tranquillizers, sleeping pills, anti-depressants and other mind-altering medications. These often have unpleasant side-effects, and frequently lead to dependency or addiction. Symptoms often return when a drug is stopped.

Other approaches, such as analysis, behavioural retraining, counselling, and techniques of encouraging emotional release, are now gaining in popularity. Some of these methods can be very helpful, but many are limited in their long-term benefits because they lack a truly wholistic understanding of mental health.

A wider macroscopic view adds a very deep and profound way of increasing our emotional and mental health. In the widest view, we must look back in time at the evolution of the human mind and consciousness as we know it, and understand the factors that have created it. Mystery still surrounds the fact that about 500,000 years ago, during the process of evolution from our ape-like ancestors, the human brain suddenly began to expand rapidly. The solution lies in a much overlooked influence on evolution, that of food. We are daily recreated by our food, it becomes our blood, our body, and our brain. At some time in our history, the diet of our ancestors turned to the seeds of grasses, or grains, as a staple food, supplemented by other vegetables, fruits and small amounts of fish or meat. The evidence for this is still with us in our teeth. Of our thirty-two teeth, twenty are the flat molars and pre-molars which are found in all plant-eating animals like cows and sheep. They are used for grinding grains, vegetables, and other plant foods. Another eight are the flattened incisors, used for biting and cutting vegetable foods. Only four are canines, the teeth found in carnivorous animals like cats and dogs, and these are much reduced in size.

It is an incontrovertible fact that thousands of years ago our teeth, as well as our whole digestive system, became adapted to a primarily vegetarian diet. When grains, which are the highest evolved plant food, became the staple food, the human brain and consciousness underwent a rapid development unseen in previous ages.

This broad view of our evolution indicates that the only way to continue our mental development is by eating a grain-based vegetarian or near-vegetarian diet. It is no coincidence that all major civilizations that have arisen in the world in the last 15,000 years have been founded on such a diet. When we depart from this ancient way of eating, as modern society has done, our mentality is likely to return to a more primitive nature, limiting the full development of our human characteristics and potentials. The most important way of approaching emotional and mental problems is therefore to return to our traditional diet—that is, to the macrobiotic way of eating.

Our broader view of the human mind also includes the whole person in his or her present environment. In our education and upbringing we have been taught to look at the world through dualistic eyes. This has resulted in the common illusion that the body and mind are quite separate, just as if there was a line at the neck dividing the head from the body! This has led to emotional and mental problems being worked on in isolation, without any thought for the influence of bodily disharmony or ill-health. This division is non-existent. The body, mind and spirit are all one; they are merely different aspects of the whole person. Improving the health of the physical body is therefore a fundamental way of creating emotional and mental health. This is not to say that food and physiological health are the only factors to look at, but that they provide the fundamental basis of emotional and mental health. We can build on this firm foundation with other ways of making positive changes in our emotional and mental experience.

The effect of environment, food and physical health on the emotions and mind will be explained in more detail in a later chapter, but it is interesting to note here the experience of many people who have used the macrobiotic way of eating to relieve physical health problems, and found that they have undergone unexpected positive psychological changes. In many cases these individuals had unsuccessfully used various methods to rid themselves of unproductive attitudes and emotions, such as chronic depression, anxiety, fearfulness, paranoia or hyper-sensitivity, but experienced a fading of symptoms over a period of months simply through changes in diet and lifestyle.

This approach encourages a much more positive attitude towards problems in life. Just as outside factors like bacteria, viruses or the weather are often blamed for physical health problems, emotional and mental difficulties are often blamed on stress, unpleasant past experiences and other external influences. This attitude sadly often leads to the conclusion that we can do little to improve the quality of our lives. With the macroscopic view, we have new ways of approaching problems. By changing our internal physiological condition and mental outlook, we can bring about many positive changes. Through self-reflection and self-examination, and finding the *internal* causes of problems, we can make the necessary changes to return to a more harmonious and enjoyable life experience. This is a much more optimistic way of perceiving problems—that it is within our own control to solve them, so that rather than resenting or fearing difficulties, we can embrace them as challenges which act as a positive stimulus for our growth. There is no limit to our growth; it is an on-going evolution that we can continue throughout our lives.

CHAPTER THREE

YIN AND YANG

In this chapter we will look in more detail at the order present in nature, using yin and yang. Although the concept of yin and yang is quite ancient, it can still bring alive a new understanding of life for us in the modern world. Life can seem a random and chaotic affair, but with yin and yang we can see that everything happens for definite reasons, following clear patterns of change. They provide us with an invaluable key to finding balance and harmony in our lives, and to creating health, happiness, and the freedom to choose our own direction in life.

Using yin and yang can also unify all branches of study and all aspects of life, because everything in nature follows the same orderly patterns. Modern thinking has divided life up into science, art, religion, medicine, astrology and so on but, with the order of the universe as a guide, one can understand how these all relate to one another. We can see the connection between the body and the mind, between the scientific study of matter and the religious study of spirituality, and between food and our physical health, moods and emotions, behaviour and thinking.

THE SYMMETRY OF NATURE

Everything in nature and the universe is inter-connected, and forms a unified whole. Within this whole, everything is divided into two opposite qualities—day and night, winter and summer, light and dark, love and hate, attraction and repulsion, sadness and joy, depression and elation. Our behaviour may be more outgoing and extrovert, or inward-looking and introvert. Our attitudes may be more conservative or liberal, materialistic or spiritual. Sometimes we are serious, at other times more light-hearted!

This scheme is shown in the well known Taoist symbol shown below:

The outer circle represents the whole, divided into two symmetrical halves, called yin and yang, which create all the opposite qualities we find in our world. Yin is the name given to energy or movement that is expanding, and can be represented as:

Yang is the name given to energy of movement that is contracting, and can be represented as:

A clear example of how these two tendencies create opposite qualities is the different form of plants and animals. Plants are stationary while animals move about. Plants convert carbon dioxide to oxygen with the green pigment chlorophyll, while animals convert oxygen to carbon dioxide, based on the red pigment haemoglobin. Plants grow their roots outwards into the soil, while we carry our 'roots' internally in the intestine where nutrients are absorbed. The respiratory system of plants, their leaves, expand upwards and outwards, while our lungs are contracted and internal. So plants are created more by the yin tendency, and animals more by the yang tendency.

By looking at the yin and yang qualities of plants, foods, or individuals, we can learn how to achieve balance and health in the body and in life. A few more examples of yin and yang will be useful in this.

We recognize two qualities of temperature, hot and cold. Heat is produced by contraction, as when air is compressed pumping up a bicycle or car tyre, and so is yang. Coolness is produced by expansion, as when liquid released from an aerosol can expands to a gas, and so is yin. The warmer colours of red, orange and yellow are therefore more yang, and the cooler colours of green, blue and violet are more yin.

Our body's structure and its functions are also based on this symmetry. It is made up of the head which is smaller and harder or yang, and the body which is larger and softer or yin. The expansion and contraction of the heart pumps blood, the rise and fall of the lungs causes breathing, and the contraction and relaxation of the intestines moves food through the digestive system.

There are two basic aspects to our thinking, which are controlled by the two halves of the brain. The left side carries out various work of a more contractive or yang nature such as analytical, logical, rational thought, and is used in more scientific and tangible activities. The right side carries out more yin work such as intuitive and synthetic thinking, and is used more in artistic and intangible activities.

FURTHER FEATURES OF YIN AND YANG

An important aspect of yin and yang for us on planet Earth is their direction of movement. The yang force comes from the sun, moon, planets, stars and outer space in the form of light, other electromagnetic radiations, and cosmic rays, moving to the earth's centre. The yin force is produced by the rotation of the earth, and moves from its centre outwards. In some cultures the yang force has therefore been called heaven's force or father, and the yin force has been called Earth's force or mother. At the surface of the earth the yang force therefore moves downwards, and the yin force upwards. The growth of plants clearly shows this. A sprouting seed on the surface of the soil sends a root downwards and a leafy shoot upwards. The root is formed more by the descending yang force, and so becomes compact and hard, while the shoot is formed more by the rising yin force, producing expanded leaves and flowers. This is illustrated in figure 3.

All these pairs of qualities are not only *opposite*, but also *complementary*, working together in harmony. For example, plants and animals depend on one another for their existence. While plants take in carbon dioxide and give out oxygen, animals take in oxygen and give out carbon dioxide,

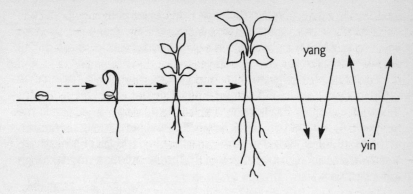

Figure 3. *The growth of plants is determined by the direction of yin and yang at the earth's surface.*

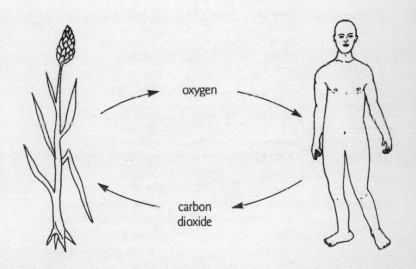

Figure 4. *The complementary exchange of gases between plants and animals.*

as shown in figure 4. When the heart beats, expansion and contraction together effectively pump the blood. Both the male and female sexes are necessary to create new life. Without experiencing sickness, we cannot appreciate what it is to be healthy.

In nature and in Man, there are many cycles created by an alternation of yin and yang, such as the seasons, the daily of cycle of night and day, the lunar cycle and the tides, cycles between opposite emotions, and between life and death. Different cycles take different lengths of time: the cycle of the seasons takes one year, the rise and fall of civilizations takes many years, while change to an opposite emotion may take only a few seconds.

	Yin	Yang
Tendency	expansion	contraction
Activity	less active	more active
Vibration	shorter wave	longer wave
Colour	violet—blue—green—yellow—orange—red	
Direction	upwards	downwards
Weight	lighter	heavier
Temperature	cooler	hotter
Light	darker	brighter
Humidity	more wet	more dry
Density	less	greater
Size	larger	smaller
Shape	expanded, more elongated	contracted, more rounded
Texture	softer	harder
Atomic particle	electron	proton
Elements	O, N, K, P, Ca	Na, H, C, Mg
Life form	plants	animals
Sex	female	male
Organ structure	hollow, e.g. bladder	solid, e.g. liver
Nerves	sympathetic system	parasympathetic system
Activity	more mental, spiritual	more physical, social
Attitude	gentle, receptive	active, outward going
Dimension	space	time

Figure 5. *Examples of yin and yang.*

Further examples of the pairs of opposite qualities created by yin and yang are given in figure 5. At first yin and yang naturally seem a little foreign and difficult to grasp, but as one applies them to more and more aspects of life they really come alive. We will be looking at some more ways of using yin and yang in the rest of this book.

CHAPTER FOUR

THE BENEFITS OF BALANCE

With an understanding of yin and yang, we can now look at the benefits of eating a diet in which these two tendencies are balanced. First, we will take a simple look at the yin and yang quality of different foods, and then consider the benefits of eating those foods which have a more balanced nature.

YIN AND YANG IN FOODS

We have already seen that animals are more yang than plants, so the first principle we can see is that *animal foods like meat, poultry, eggs and fish are more yang than plant foods like grains, vegetables, seeds, nuts and fruit.* Another principle is that *plant extracts or derivatives are usually more yin than the plants they are taken from.* This includes sugar, syrups, tea, coffee, alcohol, fruit juices and most drugs and medications. We now have three broad categories of foods, more yang animal foods, more yin plant extracts, and plant foods which fall in between.

Dairy foods do not obviously fit into these three categories, but generally hard salty cheeses have a similar quality to animal foods, and softer, lighter dairy foods like milk, yogurt and cream fall into the yin plant extract category. There is also refined salt, not a biological food but a mineral, which has a strong contractive quality and is therefore in the more yang category. The three categories are shown in figure 6.

This is a simple, common-sense way of understanding the quality of foods, which we already unconsciously know. A universal law of yin and yang is that opposites are attracted to each other, like the attraction between the positive and negative poles of a magnet, or between male and female. This law also governs our appetite, so if we eat a yang food, we are

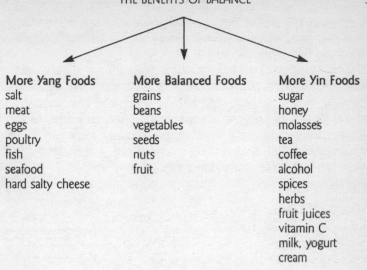

More Yang Foods
salt
meat
eggs
poultry
fish
seafood
hard salty cheese

More Balanced Foods
grains
beans
vegetables
seeds
nuts
fruit

More Yin Foods
sugar
honey
molasses
tea
coffee
alcohol
spices
herbs
fruit juices
vitamin C
milk, yogurt
cream

Figure 6. *Foods categorized by their yin and yang nature.*

automatically attracted to eating a yin food to make balance, and vice versa. For example, drinking alcohol can lead to eating salty nuts or crisps, which then increases the thirst for more alcohol.

This natural attraction has led to some interesting traditional ways of combining foods. Different meats are traditionally served with an accompaniment from the more yin category, such as mint sauce with lamb, apple sauce with pork, and horseradish with beef. Spicy and sugary sauces are favourites on eggs, sausages and beefburgers. Pickles are often eaten with cheese. Anyone who eats a lot of meat always takes a fair amount of sugar, alcohol, tea or other more yin food. If you observe the foods you are eating, you can watch your appetite swing from more yang foods to more yin foods and back again.

Many of the diets that have become fashionable in recent years have come about because of this law of attraction. Since the war, people have consumed larger amounts of meat, eggs and poultry than before. This has created an attraction to diets containing more of the yin foods, including diets low in salt, diets high in fruits and fruit juices, diets based on raw foods which have a lighter and more expansive nature than cooked foods, honey, vitamin C tablets and some other dietary supplements. Many of these diets are a reaction to past eating but, as we shall see, are not necessarily healthy in the long run.

A basic principle of the macrobiotic way of eating is to mainly choose foods from the *central, balanced category*. This creates balance and health physically, emotionally and mentally. To understand this in more detail we can look at the physical, emotional and mental effects of eating predominantly more yang foods, predominantly more yin foods, a combination of both these extremes, and of eating the balanced foods. These effects are summarized in figure 7.

Quality of Food	Our Physical, Emotional and Mental Condition
More yang	overly yang
More yin	overly yin
Both more yang and more yin	extreme yang and yin
Balanced	balanced

Figure 7. *The effects of different foods on our condition.*

BENEFITS OF PHYSICAL BALANCE

If you eat a large amount of more yang foods like meat, eggs and salt, various parts of the body become *contracted and hardened*, preventing them from functioning normally. The excessive amount of saturated animal fat in these foods is well known to be the primary cause of arteriosclerosis, in which the arteries of the heart and body become coated in fatty material, with subsequent thickening and hardening of the artery walls. Less blood can flow through these arteries and this frequently causes heart attacks and other circulatory problems. Another example is the role of excessive salt intake in causing high blood pressure. The salt causes many small arteries throughout the body to contract, so that less blood flows through them, with a build up of blood pressure. Reducing salt intake helps to bring the blood pressure back to normal.

Eating large quantities of more yin foods like sugar, honey, spices, fruit juices and alcohol causes *expansion and weakening* in the body. Very often the intestines become loose and expanded, causing either chronic diarrhoea or constipation, the growth of diverticula, and later colitis and enteritis. Other organs, such as the tonsils, adenoids and lymph glands, become inflamed. Expansion of the cells and blood vessels of the brain brings on certain forms of headaches and migraines, which in many people's experience are brought on by wine, chocolate, sugar or other yin foods.

Eating a combination of the more extreme yin and yang foods brings about a variety of problems involving both contraction and expansion, including the formation of kidney and gall stones, most skin ailments, breast cysts, and cataracts.

A fuller list of physical problems caused by these three ways of eating is shown in figure 8.

Yang	Yin	Yang and Yin
duodenal ulcers	colitis	arteriosclerosis
hepatitis	enteritis	gall bladder stones
appendicitis	hernia	kidney stones
jaundice	diabetes	arthritis
gout	asthma	breast cysts and cancer
liver cancer	pleurisy	lung cancer
headache at the back	leukaemia	cataracts
of the head	meningitis	pneumonia
	detached retina	
	varicose veins	
	gingivitis	
	stomach ulcers	
	cystitis	
	bleeding nose	
	headaches at the	
	front of the head	

Figure 8. *Diseases caused by eating imbalanced diets.*

By eating a balanced diet made up of the central category of foods, it is possible to avoid suffering from all these types of illness. If you keep eating a balanced diet, a corresponding balance is created at deeper and deeper levels of the body. The food is first absorbed by the blood, so it is here that balance first occurs, between acid and alkaline, sodium and potassium, and the levels of many other chemicals. The cells are fed by the blood, so the cells are the next level to come into balance. After this, various hormones with opposite effects, and the nervous system come into balance.

As balance penetrates to deeper levels of the body over weeks, months and years, one gains greater and greater health benefits. Apart from avoiding serious sickness, many other benefits are commonly found. The level of vitality and energy increases, allowing a fuller and more interesting life. Sleep tends to become deeper and more restful, and at the same time shorter. Body weight returns to its natural level, without efforts at counting calories and restricting one's intake of food. The body becomes more flexible, with greater stamina. Various minor health problems such as poor circulation, frequent colds and infections, blocked sinuses and ears, headaches, and sore throats disappear. And there are the emotional and mental benefits, to which we shall now turn.

EMOTIONAL BALANCE

A person functions as a whole, so that any disharmony at the physical level will also manifest itself in his or her moods and emotions. Eating predominantly more yang foods causes *energy to concentrate deep in the body*, which is often experienced as deep tension. This can produce a need to be always working and busy, and difficulty in relaxing. These people often appear to be uptight, and give the feeling of being 'bottled up'. They frequently keep a tight control over themselves, other people and situations. Often they repress or deny their feelings and emotions, preferring to use logical, intellectual thought. The bottled-up energy frequently escapes as sudden outbursts of impatience, irritability or anger. They often keep a tight hold on material possessions and money, and find it difficult to give out to other people. In the extreme, the over-consumption of yang foods can cause severe emotional disturbances including paranoia.

Eating predominantly more yin foods brings about the opposite types of moods and emotions. Expansion of the body *moves energy to the surface of the body*, which can be experienced as surface tension or nervousness, anxiety, over-excitability and over-emotional behaviour. These people frequently feel fearful and worry a lot, feel self-pity, or have a cynical and suspicious outlook. In the extreme, this can lead to problems like schizophrenia.

Eating a combination of the extreme yin and yang foods can lead to a combination of the extreme yang and yin moods and emotions, and frequent swings between these opposites.

As the benefits of eating a balanced diet progress deeper physically, they also progress to deeper levels of our moods and emotions. When one's condition has become overly yin or yang, one can be trapped in certain feelings which can be difficult to get out of just through conscious effort or by using techniques for emotional release and change. As one becomes physically balanced, old habitual moods and emotions often fall effortlessly away. This does not mean that food is the only factor in our change, but that creating balance and smooth functioning in the body creates a sound basis for a well-balanced, positive and happy emotional life, when accompanied by a positive commitment to make changes for the better. Some of the common changes experienced by people who have begun eating macrobiotically are given in figure 9.

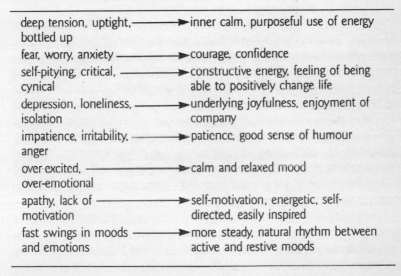

deep tension, uptight, bottled up ⟶ inner calm, purposeful use of energy

fear, worry, anxiety ⟶ courage, confidence

self-pitying, critical, cynical ⟶ constructive energy, feeling of being able to positively change life

depression, loneliness, isolation ⟶ underlying joyfulness, enjoyment of company

impatience, irritability, anger ⟶ patience, good sense of humour

over-excited, over-emotional ⟶ calm and relaxed mood

apathy, lack of motivation ⟶ self-motivation, energetic, self-directed, easily inspired

fast swings in moods and emotions ⟶ more steady, natural rhythm between active and restive moods

Figure 9. *Common changes experienced by people eating a balanced macrobiotic diet.*

MENTAL BALANCE

When our condition becomes overly yang or yin, our expression and thinking are also affected. An overly yang condition is characterized by *hardness and inflexibility*. This can manifest itself as rigidity, stubbornness, and an inability to see points of view other than their own. They frequently feel superior to others, and are over-confident, domineering, and exclude other people.

An overly yin condition is characterized by a *loose or spaced out mentality*. These people have difficulty in concentrating on one subject or task, and life often lacks direction and purposefulness. Thinking is vague and impractical, and divorced from action, so that daydreams go unrealized. Money and opportunities frequently slip through their hands.

Most people have consumed a fair amount of both extremes of yin and yang foods, and so experience a mixture of these characteristics. However, most people fall clearly into one or other category. If you think of yourself and people you know, it will become quite easy to see examples of overly yin and yang expression and thinking. Some further examples of typical characteristics are shown in figure 10.

As the internal balance gained from eating a balanced diet reaches the hormonal and nervous system, these opposite ways of thinking tend to diminish and be replaced by more balanced behaviour and thinking. This transformation can be greatly aided by consciously achieving greater balance. For example, you realize that you are neither superior or inferior to other people, but of equal worth. Instead of excluding or depending on other people, you can embrace all people without leaning on them. While having your own firm views, you can be open to new ideas from other people and to changing your own views. A balance can be reached between attending to the material and spiritual aspects of life in a unified way. Rather than existing mainly in past memories or future plans, you can enjoy the present moment.

These extreme ways of expression and thinking are all delusions, for they do not exist in reality, but are merely the result of an imbalanced physiological condition. Harmonizing the opposite forces of yin and yang in your whole being therefore opens the door to a new level of existence. You can go beyond dealing primarily with your physical, emotional and mental difficulties and conflicts, and reach a deeper awareness of yourself.

	Overly Yang	Overly Yin
Expression	domineering	submissive
	insensitivity to others	over-sensitive
	aggressive	defensive
	over-confident	under-confident
	self-assertive	self-denying
	exclusion of others	dependency on others
Attitudes and Thinking	stubborn, dogmatic	lack of conviction or firm views
	too grounded, materialistic	up in the air, impractical
	inability to appreciate other's views	overly impressionable
	obsessed by order	lack of orderliness
	overly concerned with past	overly concerned with future
	denial of philosophical and spiritual aspects of live	denial of practical and material aspects of life

Figure 10. *Mental tendencies produced by an overly yang and overly yin condition.*

You can discover the true potential that you have been given to use and express in this lifetime, including an unending source of joy and love for people and life. After eating the balanced macrobiotic diet for some time, many people realize what it is they really want to do in their lives, and feel the energy and motivation to begin on this new path. With clearer thinking and a growing sense of intuition, you can get into the flow of your life, unimpeded by mental confusions and dilemmas. This is the beginning of a more adventurous, creative and amusing life ahead.

CHAPTER FIVE

DESIGNING A BALANCED DIET

In the last chapter different foods were classified into three broad categories, and we saw the benefits of eating from the central balanced category. In this chapter we will look in more detail at the unique qualities of different foods, so that we can design a balanced and healthful diet for ourselves.

THE YIN AND YANG OF FOODS

To some extent, our common sense tells us whether a food is more yin or yang. More yang foods like eggs, meat and cheese feel 'heavier' and more filling, and give us a feeling of warmth. More yin foods like fruits, yogurt and spices are 'lighter' and less filling, and feel more cooling. To further develop our understanding of the yin and yang qualities of foods, we can use some specific characteristics of yin and yang foods. These are shown in figure 11.

A few examples will show more clearly how we can use these characteristics. First, compare meat with white fish. Meat is drier and darker, and comes from a warm-blooded mammal that is relatively recently evolved. The fish is moister and white, and comes from a cold-blooded animal, in a more anciently evolved group. Therefore, meat is more yang than the fish.

Next, compare a melon with rice. Rice is smaller, harder and drier. It is lower in potassium, grows in temperate climates, and is a recently evolved species. A melon is larger, softer and wetter. It is higher in potassium, and grows in warmer environments, and as a fruit is a more ancient type of food. Rice is therefore more yang than melon.

These characteristics can also be used to compare different varieties within the major food groups of fish, grains, vegetables, fruits and so

	Yang	Yin
ANIMAL AND PLANT FOODS		
Taste	bitter—salty—sweet—sour—spicy	
Water content	drier	wetter
Chemical balance	higher in sodium	higher in potassium
Size	smaller	larger
Environment	colder	warmer
Species	more modern	more ancient
ANIMAL FOODS		
Activity	faster moving	slower moving
Body temperature	higher	lower
Colour of flesh	black—red—brown—white—transparent	
Nutritional components	minerals—protein—fat	
PLANT FOODS		
Growth rate	slower	faster
Direction of growth	downwards, or growing horizontally above ground	upwards, or growing horizontally below ground
Season of growth	autumn and winter	spring and summer
Odour	less aromatic	more aromatic
Height	shorter	taller
Nutritional components	minerals—carbohydrate—protein—fat—oil	

Figure 11. *Characteristics of yang and yin foods.*

on. For example, compare rice with corn. Rice is a smaller, harder grain that grows in a cooler climate, and so is more yang than corn. Using these characteristics, various grains can be arranged from yang to yin as follows:

buckwheat—millet—short-grain rice—wheat—barley—oats—corn

In the same way, all commonly eaten foods can be arranged on a scale from yang to yin, as shown in figure 12. At first this table is a very useful guide to the yin and yang quality of different foods, but over time you will develop greater sensitivity to the yin and yang qualities of foods through

Figure 12. *A classification of foods from yang to yin.*

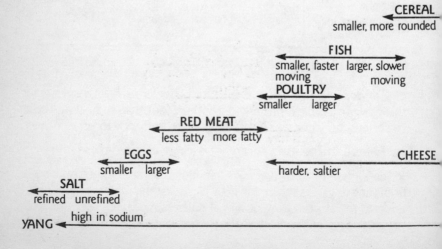

SUGAR
less refined   more refined

SPICES
less aromatic   more aromatic

STIMULANTS
eg. coffee, tea, carob, cocoa

ALCOHOLIC DRINKS
grain-based   fruit-based
less alcoholic   more alcoholic

COOKING OIL
from seeds   from nuts, fruits

FRUIT
smaller, temperate larger, tropical

NUTS
less oily   more oily

VEGETABLES
roots   round   leafy

SEEDS
smaller   larger

BEANS
smaller   larger

GRAINS
larger, more elongated

CREAM
less fatty   more fatty

YOGURT
less fatty   more fatty

MILK
less fatty   more fatty

softer, sweeter

high in potassium
YIN

their effects on your health, moods and thinking. Your own sense of the qualities of particular foods can come more and more into play, slowly replacing the intellectual use of these characteristics.

DESIGNING A BALANCED DIET

When designing a balanced diet, we should try to select foods from the central, more balanced, part of this scale: grains, beans and vegetables, with smaller amounts of fish, fruit, seeds, nuts and some other foods. The question is often asked, 'Why can't I balance meat and sugar, or eggs and honey?' The reason is that these foods are so extreme in their contractive and expansive effects, that while one organ or function in the body becomes overly contracted, another becomes overly expanded. For example, with a diet containing much meat and sugar, the stomach and liver frequently become over-contracted, while the heart and large intestine become overly expanded. In time, this will lead to various health problems, as well as creating the more extreme emotions and attitudes described in the previous chapter. These more extreme yin and yang foods are also more difficult for the body to digest and use. They thus leave excess fats or toxins for the body to discharge, placing greater stress and strain on the body.

As well as avoiding the more extreme yin and yang foods, it is wise to avoid all dairy foods including milk, butter, cheese, yogurt and cream, whether made from cow's or goat's milk. Common sense tells us that milk is the food nature designed for babies and other newborn mammals. It is an ideal food at this stage of life, rich in fats, sugars, calcium and other minerals important for quick growth. There is no good reason why it should continue to be a suitable food source after this time. In fact, only about 10 per cent of the world's adult population consumes milk and its products. On a world scale, eating dairy foods is the exception, not the norm.

Eating dairy foods produces many problems for children and adults. Its high fat content, so necessary for a rapidly growing baby, is simply not needed after the first year or two of life, and so forms fat deposits in arteries, in and around organs, and under the skin. Dairy foods are extremely mucus-forming, and are a primary cause of mucus in the lungs, sinuses and ears, especially in children. The argument that milk is necessary as a source of calcium is simply not true, as many other foods contain more by weight, including greens like kale, parsley and watercress, beans like chickpeas and soya beans, hazelnuts and almonds. Sesame seeds and many sea vegetables actually contain ten times more calcium than cow's milk.

THE STANDARD MACROBIOTIC DIET

Michio Kushi has designed a diet plan based on the more balanced foods in the central part of the yin-yang scale. This is generally suitable for people living in a temperate climate such as Great Britain, Northern Europe and North America. It is often referred to as the *Standard Macrobiotic Diet*, and is shown in figure 13.

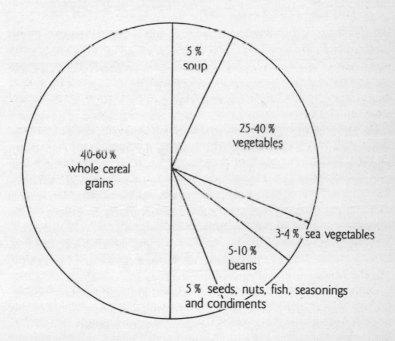

Figure 13. *The Standard Macrobiotic Diet.*

About half of the diet is made up of whole cereal grains, providing bulk and energy. These include brown rice, barley, wheat, buckwheat and corn, and various flour products made from whole grains like wholemeal bread, noodles and porridge oats. A wide variety of vegetables, prepared in many different ways, form about a quarter to a third of the diet. Sea vegetables form a small but important part, due to their high mineral and vitamin content. Beans, and a small quantity of fish if desired, provide a richer source of protein, and seeds, nuts and fruit form a small additional part of the diet. Many people's first reaction to seeing this plan is how limited it is! However, as we shall see in later chapters, it offers an endless range of appetizing meals, possibly much wider than the fare you eat at the moment.

THE YIN AND YANG OF COOKING

We have looked at how to balance yin and yang in our choice of foods. Cooking changes the yin or yang quality of a food, so we must also be aware of how to create balance in our preparation and cooking of these foods. First, we should think about why we cook foods at all as it is sometimes said that it is preferable to eat most foods raw. Common sense tells us that when living in a cold climate, cooking is desirable to create more warming food that generates heat within us. In hotter climates, less cooking is needed, so that the cooling quality of foods is retained. In our temperate climate, eating some salad and raw foods is fine in the summer, but only a small quantity is needed in the winter. Eating mainly raw foods during cold winter months often results in difficulties getting warm, colds, a general loss of vitality and other problems caused by the expansion and cooling of the body.

It is also sometimes said that cooking destroys minerals and vitamins. However, minerals cannot be destroyed at the temperatures used in cooking, and the only vitamin that can be broken down by normal cooking times is vitamin C, which is destroyed by approximately ten minutes of boiling. For this reason, green vegetables, which contain large amounts of this vitamin, should usually only be lightly steamed or boiled.

It is also frequently said that cooking will kill food, and destroy its life force. This life force is actually a dynamic interaction of the yin and yang energy in plants. If you use your knowledge of yin and yang in cooking, this dynamic interaction can be increased to give you a greater charge of energy from your food, rather than diminishing it. When you eat only uncooked foods, you are also subservient to your environment and the foods available in it. The skill of cooking with a knowledge of yin and yang gives you the ability to adapt to different environments and activities, and to freely control your health and destiny.

The type of heat you choose to cook your food has a large effect on your health. Various types of heat have been used in cooking at different times in our history. Wood and charcoal were the earliest sources of heat, and more recently coal, gas and electricity have come into use. In the past decade, microwaves have become increasingly popular. To help you understand the effects of these different types of heat, they can be arranged on a scale from yang to yin as follows:

wood
charcoal
coal
gas
electricity
microwave

Any of the more yang types of heat from wood to gas can be used to produce a healthy balance in the body. Electric cooking over a long period of time will create an overly yin, weakened condition. It is particularly advisable for people suffering from illnesses to use a more yang type of heat than electricity to give them strength to aid their recovery. The regular use of microwave cooking can create an even weaker physical and mental condition, so it is advisable to avoid using it too frequently.

We must also be aware of how different methods of cooking change the quality of foods. Cooking uses various elements. Some of these make food more yang, such as heat, salt and pressure. Others make food more yin, including fermentation and adding vinegar, mustard, ginger or more water. The more yang elements we use the more yang foods become, and using more yin elements will make food more yin. We can therefore arrange different cooking methods from yang to yin as follows:

deep-frying
baking
pressure cooking

stir-frying
steaming
boiling
pickling
pressing salads
raw salads

When creating balanced meals, the more balanced cooking methods should be used more often, and the more strongly yin and yang methods less often. Pressure cooking, stir-frying, boiling and steaming can all be used daily, and deep-fried, baked, pickled, pressed and raw salads used less often or in smaller amounts.

Dishes should be kept simple, with relatively few ingredients and seasonings, and with the minimum amount of interference through over-frequent stirring or mixing. This allows the unique quality of each food to come through clearly in a meal. If many ingredients are combined in one dish without discretion, you will receive a confusion of many different energies from it. It can be tempting to throw a lot of different things into a dish to make sure that it is attractive and flavoursome, but as your cooking of macrobiotic meals improves, you will be able to produce the most appetizing dishes by combining only a few well-chosen ingredients in a well-prepared manner.

Preparing balanced, healthful and appetizing meals is a great art, which is important if you are to get the best from your food. It is really something like alchemy—taking basic ingredients and using the elements of cooking to create the greatest physical, psychological and spiritual health in those eating the food. Like all arts, it can give great pleasure and satisfaction, and can be a lot of fun.

THE MACROBIOTIC DIET IN PERSPECTIVE

There has been a lot of interest in eating more healthily in recent years, with many people making beneficial changes to their diets. This growing interest has come mainly from individuals wanting a healthier way of living, but is increasingly being supported by scientific research. In 1983 the British government published the report, *Proposals for Nutritional Guidelines for Health Education in Britain*, often called the NACNE report as it was prepared for the National Advisory Committee on Nutrition

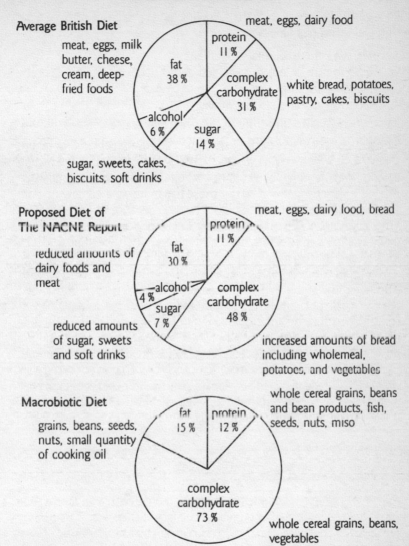

Average British Diet

meat, eggs, milk
butter, cheese,
cream, deep-
fried foods

meat, eggs, dairy food

protein 11%

fat 38%

complex carbohydrate 31%

white bread, potatoes,
pastry, cakes, biscuits

alcohol 6%

sugar 14%

sugar, sweets, cakes,
biscuits, soft drinks

**Proposed Diet of
The NACNE Report**

reduced amounts of
dairy foods and
meat

meat, eggs, dairy food, bread

protein 11%

fat 30%

alcohol 4%

sugar 7%

complex carbohydrate 48%

reduced amounts
of sugar, sweets
and soft drinks

increased amounts of bread
including wholemeal,
potatoes, and vegetables

Macrobiotic Diet

grains, beans, seeds,
nuts, small quantity
of cooking oil

whole cereal grains, beans
and bean products, fish,
seeds, nuts, miso

fat 15%

protein 12%

complex carbohydrate 73%

whole cereal grains, beans,
vegetables

Figure 14. *The nutritional profile of the average British diet, the proposed diet of the NACNE report, and the macrobiotic diet (percentages are of total energy intake) with the main sources of these nutrients.*

Education. The report made the following long-term proposals to reduce the level of serious illnesses:

1. *Reducing* the total intake of all fats.
2. *Reducing* the intake of saturated animal fats.
3. *Reducing* sugar intake.
4. *Reducing* salt and alcohol intake.
5. *Increasing* the consumption of whole grains, vegetables and fruit.

Similar suggestions were made by the American government in their report, *Dietary Goals for the United States*, published in 1977. It is interesting to note that the original recommendations of both reports suggested making larger changes in diet, but these had to be watered down before they were allowed to be published. This was because of pressure from other government departments and big food-producing businesses. Thus many scientists and doctors feel that there is enough scientific evidence for advising much greater changes in diet in order to reduce disease.

How does the macrobiotic diet fit into this general movement towards a healthier way of eating? Figure 14 compares today's average British diet, the proposals of the NACNE report, and a typical macrobiotic diet. It can be seen that the macrobiotic way of eating carries the scientific proposals another step. It contains virtually no saturated animal fat, and the minimum of total fats. It completely avoids the use of sugar. Through using whole, natural foods it almost completely avoids having to eat artificial chemicals and additives. It also increases the health benefits of food with its principle of balance, and with its well-established cooking methods it offers an endless variety of nutritious and appetizing dishes and meals.

CHAPTER SIX

WHAT TO EAT

In the last chapter we looked at the Standard Macrobiotic Diet, which is a general plan for a healthy and balanced way of eating. In this chapter we will take a closer look at each of the food categories in the Standard Diet, discussing their nutritional value and how to use them.

CEREAL GRAINS

Thousands of years ago our ancestors began eating grains, and almost every major culture in the world has used them as their staple food. In ancient China, people ate millet, rice and buckwheat; in India, rice and wheat; in the Middle East, wheat and barley; in parts of Africa, sorghum; in northern and central America, corn; and in Northern Europe wheat, barley, rye and oats. The importance of grains in the history of our culture is revealed in the word *meal*, which simply means *ground grain*, and in the names of the family provider as the *bread winner* and of money as *bread*. The Lord's prayer begins with the line, *Give us this day our daily bread*. Clearly, grains were a central part of life to our ancestors, in a diet very different to the modern diet in which they form only a small part.

The best way to eat grains on a regular basis is in their whole form, such as short or medium-grain rice, pot or pearl barley, wheat, millet, sweet rice, buckwheat and corn. Flour products made from whole grains can also be used, but in smaller quantities. These include wholewheat or buckwheat noodles, various kinds of wholewheat pasta and spaghetti, cous-cous, bulgar wheat, steel-cut or rolled oats and other grains, corn grits and corn meal, pastry and bread. It is not good to eat these flour products too often as the splitting of whole grains into fragments causes some of their vital energy to be lost, and once broken open some of their nutritional components begin to decompose. Whole grains are also very easily digested, whereas flour products are more difficult to digest, as well as being more acid-forming in the stomach and mucus-forming in the whole body.

Grains make up 40-60 per cent of the diet, and are eaten at almost every meal. Generally, the grain portion of a meal should be a whole grain, with flour products kept as occasional additions or as snacks and in desserts.

The best form of bread to eat is natural rise or *sourdough*. This is the oldest method of bread-making. If you cannot buy sourdough bread, you can make it by mixing some wholemeal flour in water and allowing it to ferment until sour. This 'starter' is then kneaded with the bread dough, and allowed to rise naturally for 12-20 hours before being baked. Sourdough bread is far more digestible because of the pre-digestion of the flour by the natural micro-organisms living on grains. It also has a beautifully sweet taste, quite unlike yeasted bread. This method of bread-making also avoids adding artificial yeasts, which are excessively yin, as can be seen from their effect of producing the very rapid rising and expansion of bread dough. It should be noted that baking whole grains into bread generally makes them drier and harder, or more yang. Using bread as your main form of grain will therefore tend to make you drier and more yang.

VEGETABLES

Vegetables make up 25-40 per cent of the diet, providing a great variety of colours, tastes and textures, and many different vitamins and minerals. To obtain a balance between yin and yang and different minerals and vitamins, a wide variety of vegetables should be used regularly, including leafy greens, round and root vegetables.

Greens include spring cabbage, kale, leeks, broccoli, Chinese cabbage, watercress, spring onions (scallions), bok choy, Brussels sprouts, dandelion greens, parsley and turnip greens. Green vegetables are an important source of vitamins A and C. It is widely believed that it is necessary to eat large quantities of fruit to obtain vitamin C, but in fact a cup of greens like broccoli or kale contains more of the vitamin than an orange.

Round vegetables include onions, swede (rutabaga), turnips, green and orange pumpkins and cabbage. They are an excellent source of natural sweetness when they are well cooked.

Root vegetables include carrots, parsnips, burdock, salsify, and daikon (also called mooli or long white radish). Together with some of the round varieties, roots are rich in complex carbohydrates as well as minerals and vitamins. They therefore need greater digestive effort, which in turn produces warmth. This makes them particularly good in the winter.

Vegetables can be cooked in many different ways and in different combinations to give a great variety of appearances and tastes. These include boiling, steaming, stir-frying, baking, pressure-cooking, in stews, casseroles and soups, and as pickles and salads. In our temperate climate it is generally best to eat about three-quarters of vegetables cooked, and a quarter as pickles and salad.

It is best to use fresh vegetables, either from your own garden or from a good greengrocer's shop. Organic vegetables are becoming increasingly available in shops, and are obviously preferable as they do not contain chemical fertilizers, pesticides, herbicides, or fungicides. It is also a good idea to use as much of a vegetable as possible. They are created whole, with their own balance of nutrients, and the more of the vegetable you eat the more you benefit from the variety and balance of nutrients that it contains. You can leave the skins on round and root vegetables, and just scrub them clean with a stiff brush. If you can buy turnips, radishes, carrots, cauliflowers or leeks with their full leaves on, these can be used as well.

SEA VEGETABLES

These seem like a strange food to many people, but you have almost certainly already eaten large amounts of them! Many prepared foods, especially those that include a thickener, such as ice cream, puddings, and many dressings and cheeses, contain carrageen, algin or agar. In fact, sea vegetables have been eaten for centuries by many peoples around the world. Some examples are Irish moss and carrageen in Ireland, laver bread in Wales, and dulse and sweet kelp in Scotland and England.

Sea vegetables are an important part of the macrobiotic diet as they contain high levels of many nutrients. For example, kelp has 150 times more iodine than any land vegetable, and eight times more magnesium. Dulse has 200 times more iron than beet greens, the richest land vegetable. Hiziki, a dark sea vegetable, has fourteen times more calcium than cow's milk. As a group, they are also high in vitamins A, B, B_{12}, C and E.

Many varieties are now available in a dried form, which will keep for months. These include kelp, kombu, arame, dulse, hiziki, Irish moss, nori (laver), wakame and agar-agar. They form 3-4 per cent of the diet and are used in a variety of ways. Dulse and wakame can be used in soups; kombu, kelp or wakame can be cooked with beans and in stews; arame and hiziki can be prepared with vegetables, and the flat sheets of nori can be wrapped around balls of rice or used to make Japanese sushi. Agar-agar is used as a setting agent for making jellies.

Because sea vegetables add minerals to food, you will find that using them in bean and vegetable dishes really brings out the flavour of the other ingredients. If you find their taste difficult to take at first, begin by using them in dishes where they tend to disappear, such as wakame or dulse cooked for 20-30 minutes in a soup or stew.

BEANS AND BEAN PRODUCTS

Beans and their products are staging a come-back after some years of neglect—apart from the ever-popular baked beans of course! Along with grains, they formed an important part of many traditional diets around the world, until increased use of meat, poultry and dairy foods replaced them. They provide a concentrated source of protein, as well as vitamins and minerals like calcium, iron and vitamin B. Their protein is superior to that of meat as it is more easily digested, and does not contain the saturated animal fats that inevitably come with meat and dairy foods.

When beans are used as part of a diet along with grains, the protein from the two foods complement each other. Both beans and grains are low in a few amino acids necessary for our body, but each contains the amino acids that the other lacks. Together, these two foods supply most of the protein in the macrobiotic diet.

Many types of beans and pulses, such as aduki beans, chickpeas, green or brown lentils, kidney beans, black-eye beans, black and yellow soya beans, haricot beans and split peas can be used. There are also several foods made from soya beans, including tofu (soya bean curd), tempeh (cakes of fermented soya beans), and soya milk. Tofu and tempeh have been used in China and the Far East for centuries, and add a very different taste and texture to one's diet. Tempeh is also an excellent source of vitamin B_{12}. Soya milk is an extract of the more yin elements of soya beans, and is too yin to use on a regular basis, although it can be a very useful substitute when you are just beginning to cut out cow's milk.

Beans and bean products form 5-10 per cent of the macrobiotic diet, which works out at about 1-2 heaped tablespoons a day. There are many ways of preparing them, but it is generally good to cook them with a small amount of sea vegetable. The high mineral content of sea vegetables balances the high protein content of the beans, and makes them easier to digest. If you get wind from eating beans, this could be the answer!

SOUPS

Soups are an excellent addition to your daily fare, and can be made with a wide variety of vegetables, beans, grains and sea vegetables. They can be seasoned with sea salt, shoyu (a good quality soy sauce) or miso. It is especially good to use miso on a regular basis. Miso is a dark paste, made by fermenting soya beans with sea salt, and often a grain like barley, wheat or rice. As with tempeh, it provides vitamin B_{12}, and is a good source of easily digested protein. If you can get an unpasteurized miso, it will also provide live enzymes that aid digestion and promote bowel health. A small quantity can be added to almost any soup, giving a rich, full flavour.

SEEDS AND NUTS

A small amount of seeds and nuts provide a crunchy and tasty part of the diet, and are nutritious as well. In particular, they contain a large amount of fat in a natural form, and sesame seeds contain ten times as much calcium as cow's milk. Their high fat content makes them a little difficult to digest. Lightly roasting them in a dry frying pan, under the grill, or in the oven makes them more digestible, as well as enhancing their flavour.

Varieties to use include sesame, pumpkin and sunflower seeds, and almonds, chestnuts, peanuts, walnuts and hazelnuts. These can be eaten as a tasty snack, or combined with grains, vegetables, breads, and in desserts. Because of their high fat content it is advisable to limit their use to two or three handfuls a week. Seed and nut butters like sunflower spread, tahini and peanut butter can also be used, but in small quantities only due to their oily nature.

FRUIT

Fruit is towards the yin end of the yin-yang scale of foods, and so forms only a small part of the Standard Diet. Generally, a small quantity two to four times a week is plenty. For a person with an overly yin condition it may be advisable to eat less than this. This seems opposite to many people's advice, which is to eat as much fruit as possible. However, as we saw in the last chapter, this is generally a reaction to eating a lot of yang foods like salt, eggs, meat, hard cheeses and wholemeal bread. Watery fruits high in potassium provide a crude balance for these foods, but when you begin eating more of the central balanced foods your need for fruits will diminish. It is often said that we need lots of fruit for vitamin C but, as we have already seen, many greens contain more of this vitamin, without having the strong expansive effect of fruit.

Varieties for regular use include apples, pears, apricots, cherries, peaches, plums, strawberries, blackberries, redcurrants, grapes, raspberries, canteloupe and water melon. Dried fruits, such as sultanas, raisins, currants, apple rings and Hunza apricots (very sweet!), can also be used. They are best eaten cooked in desserts, but can sometimes be eaten raw, especially on hot summer days.

FISH AND SEAFOOD

Fish and seafood can form a small part of the macrobiotic diet, say once or twice a week, but for many people they are not an essential food and some people choose not to eat them at all. They have several advantages over other kinds of animal food. They provide protein which is more easily digested than that of meat, poultry, eggs and dairy foods, and with much less saturated animal fat. If one chooses fresh fish and seafood, they will not contain the artificial hormones, antibiotics, preservatives and colourings that other meats and dairy foods contain.

As fish is one of the most yang groups in the macrobiotic diet, it is best to choose the more yin white-fleshed varieties, which are also generally lower in fat. These include cod, haddock, plaice, flounder, bass, sole, coley, trout and dab. The sedentary seafoods like clams, oysters, mussels and cockles are the most yin of seafoods, and can also be used. The more active and yang species like shrimps, prawns, crab and lobsters can also be eaten occasionally.

SEASONINGS AND CONDIMENTS

The use of seasonings in cooking and the addition of condiments to food are important in improving the digestibility of some dishes and adding a variety of flavours. Some are more yang, such as salt, miso, tamari, shoyu soy sauce and umeboshi (pickled plums). Others are more yin, like vinegar, ginger, mustard and horseradish. We can look at the yang ones first.

Sea Salt

In the past few years there has been some controversy over the use of salt. It has been found that its over-use causes many problems, including high blood pressure, and contributes to the hardening of arteries. This has led some people to advise that we use none at all. Certainly many people do use far too much of this very yang food, and could benefit from not using any for a limited period. However, for most people a small quantity is desirable to provide sodium and minerals that are necessary for the proper functioning of the blood, muscles, nerves and other systems of the body. A small amount can be used in cooking to enhance the flavour of foods and aid digestion, but dishes should not generally taste salty. Used in this way salt combines with foods and is slowly released in digestion. It should not be added to food at the table, when it will be quickly absorbed by the body.

Of the various kinds of salt available, sea salt is the most balanced and suitable. Common salt is highly refined and is almost entirely made up of sodium chloride, whereas sea salt also contains up to 5 per cent of naturally occurring potassium, calcium, magnesium, iodine, and other trace elements. These more yin elements make sea salt more yin than common salt, and give it its mild flavour and good taste.

Of all our foods, salt is probably the most difficult to learn to take at the correct level. If too much is used, one becomes more yang. Common signs of over-use include becoming unduly thirsty after meals, retaining excess liquid in the body, a tendency to over-eat, and an attraction to lots of yin foods like fruits, sweets and alcohol. Emotionally, one tends to become tight, tense and irritable. Using too little salt can result in one becoming too yin, with signs like a lack of muscle tone, physical weakness and sluggish circulation. Mentally, it can produce 'spaciness' and a lack of alertness and concentration. You may notice other signs of consuming too much or too little salt, so experiment and find your optimum level.

Miso, Tamari, Shoyu Soy Sauce

It has already been mentioned that miso is produced by the fermentation of soya beans with sea salt. Genuine tamari is the liquid drained off during the process of making miso, and has a thick, strong flavour. Shoyu is a traditionally made soy sauce commonly produced by the fermentation of soya beans with sea salt and wheat. You should make sure that you use shoyu rather than other kinds of soy sauce, which frequently contain sugar and artificial colourings, flavourings and preservatives.

Miso paste can be used to season soups, stews, gravies, sauces, salad dressings and other dishes. Tamari and shoyu can often be used instead of sea salt, adding a delightful flavour to many dishes. Care should be taken not to use too much, though, as they contain 10-20 per cent salt.

Umeboshi

Umeboshi are green plums pickled in sea salt, with a unique sour and salty taste. They can be used to flavour sauces and salad dressings, and are also very useful as a home remedy. They are highly alkalizing and can be used to combat over-acidity in the stomach. The lactic acid they contain can help intestinal gas and poor digestion by neutralizing harmful micro-organisms.

Vinegar

Commercially-made vinegar is very acid, and usually contains chemical additives. The least acidic and most healthful type to use is rice vinegar, followed by cider vinegar. A little of these vinegars can be used over vegetables and in dressings and sauces to add a nice sharp flavour.

Ginger, Mustard, Horseradish

These can all be used in small amounts to give a hot, pungent taste to various dishes. It is best to buy root ginger rather than the powdered variety, and grate it finely before adding it to dishes. Mustard and horseradish should be pure, and not adulterated with other additives.

Condiments

Many different condiments can be used in place of salt, pepper and commercially-made sauces. A particularly healthful one is gomasio, sometimes called sesame salt. This is made by grinding 1 part of sea salt with 12 to 16 parts of toasted whole brown sesame seeds. When freshly made, it has the most amazing nutty aroma and taste. The recipe for making gomasio is given on page 151. Sesame, pumpkin and sunflower seeds can all be roasted, ground, and sprinkled over food. Other possibilities include mustard, chopped chives, parsley or spring onions, and sauerkraut and other naturally made pickles.

NATURAL SWEETENERS

As we have seen, sugar has an extreme effect on the body and mind, and should be totally avoided. This category includes other foods high in sugar like brown and demerara sugar, molasses and honey. A primary source of sweetness in the macrobiotic diet is the natural sweetness of well-cooked vegetables like onions, carrots and parsnips. Further sweetness comes from dried fruits, and using natural sweeteners like barley malt (malt extract), rice syrup, and apple juice in desserts.

OIL

Small amounts of essential oils are necessary for health, and must be present in the diet. These are mostly obtained in their natural state from grains, beans, seeds and nuts. In addition, a small quantity of good quality oil can be used for frying grains, vegetables, and other dishes. The best kinds are cold-pressed sesame and corn oil. Other types which can be used less often are olive, peanut, safflower, sunflower and soya bean oil.

Our requirement for oil is quite small, and a teaspoon of oil every day or every other day is usually adequate. It is quite possible to eat excess vegetable fats and oils, which will accumulate in the body in the same way as animal fats. For this reason, margarines do not form part of the diet, and care should be taken not to overdo the use of oil and seed and nut butters.

MACROBIOTIC SNACKS

You may sometimes feel like a snack between meals, so here are a few ideas for what you could have.

Rice cakes are made of puffed rice, and are available in most health and wholefood shops. They are especially good if you are wanting a dry biscuit-like snack. They can be eaten as they are, or with a spread like chickpea pâté or scrambled tofu. A small amount of sesame or sunflower spread could also be used occasionally.

Roasted seeds and nuts make a delicious snack. You can make up a jar at a time, so that you have always got some at hand for times when you feel like a nibble.

Home-made popcorn can be made with a little sesame oil. Take a bag for the interval when you go to the cinema, and you will be popular!

BEVERAGES

Most beverages in common use have a very yin nature. Coffee and tea contain the stimulant caffeine, and most herb teas also have a stimulating effect. Many soft drinks and juices have sugar, artificial sweeteners and various chemicals added. There are a wide range of more balanced beverages that can take their place.

The best drinks to use on a daily basis are twig or stem tea (also called Bancha or Kukicha), grain coffees like Yannoh, Barleycup and Caro, dandelion coffee, roasted barley tea, or spring or well water. Other beverages that can be used occasionally are Mu tea (a balanced blend of yin and yang herbs), apple juice, vegetable juices and non-aromatic herb teas like chamomile and lime blossom.

Alcohol is a yin substance, as you can tell from its quick evaporation, and the effects of excess on you! The fermentation of different foods to create alcoholic drinks makes those foods more yin. An alcoholic beverage will therefore be less extreme when made from a more yang food like grains, than when made from a more yin food like fruit. The distilling of spirits to increase their alcohol content also increases their yin quality. Therefore small quantities of traditionally-made beers, saki (rice wine), and whisky can be drunk occasionally, but it is better to avoid wines and other spirits.

You will find further ideas of preparing meals in chapter 14, and plenty of recipes to start you off in chapter 15.

CHAPTER SEVEN

ADAPTING THE DIET TO CHANGING NEEDS

As we have seen in previous chapters, regaining and maintaining our health depends on eating a balanced diet. How this balance is created will be different for everyone, as people's natural environment, life history and present lifestyle are all different. There can be no such thing as a diet that is suitable for everyone, everywhere, at all times. The macrobiotic understanding of healthy eating has the flexibility to allow for these differences. Using yin and yang, we can understand quite simply how to create balance for anyone, anywhere.

In this chapter we will look at how we can adapt our diet according to these changing needs. Firstly, we will consider how to make balance according to *differences in our external environment*, with the climate we live in and with the seasons. Secondly, we will look at how to make balance according to *personal differences* in age, past eating habits, and level and types of activity.

FOOD FOR DIFFERENT CLIMATES

The traditional diets of people living in different climates vary enormously, from the mostly fish and meat diet of the Eskimos, to the starchy cassava and green bananas that form the staple food in some parts of Africa. Yet many of these groups of people enjoy much better health than people who eat the more modern mixed diets. Why is this?

If we look at the plants growing in different climates, those in the colder more yin polar and sub-polar regions of the world are small and hardy, or yang. In the hotter more yang tropics, plant life reaches a much greater size and contains more water, and is therefore more yin. So plants stay in balance with the climate they grow in by evolving *an opposite and complementary structure*.

Like plants, we must adapt to local conditions to stay alive and in good health. We can do this in the same way: *in colder climates we make ourselves more yang, and in hotter climates we make ourselves more yin*. The easiest way to do this is to eat the plants and animals that are naturally available in the local environment. They are well adapted to their particular environment, so by eating them we will also become adapted to it. In a polar climate, eating the locally available fish and animal foods will make us more yang, burning to give the body a lot of heat and energy. In a tropical climate, the local plant foods with their greater cooling effect will keep us cool, and little or no animal food will be needed. In between, in a temperate climate, the Standard Macrobiotic Diet is appropriate, with local plant foods and a small amount of fish or seafood if desired.

The principle of eating local foods is based on recognizing our close relationship and dependency on our natural surroundings. It is an ecological law which all other plants and animals observe, as did our ancestors until more recent times. Practically, the more yin perishable foods like fruits and vegetables should usually come from our own region of a country, as they will not stay fresh for long. Less perishable foods like grains, beans and dried sea vegetables can come from further afield, as long as they come from a similar climate. Our most yang food, sea salt, can come from any part of the globe.

Eating by this ecological principle has several advantages. It means that we eat fresher foods, and do not need to use foods artificially preserved by canning or with chemicals. It is also more economical, both for ourselves and for the world, as transporting foods from great distances tends to be expensive.

Most readers will be living in a temperate climate, in which the most suitable grains are short and medium grain rice, barley, wheat, oats, rye, corn, and buckwheat. Long grain and basmati rice are not suitable for regular use, but could be used occasionally in the summer. Our selection of beans can include aduki beans, chickpeas, green or brown lentils, soya, kidney, haricot and black-eye beans, and split peas. Tropical varieties like butter beans are not healthful. Most traditionally-grown local vegetables can be eaten, but not potatoes, tomatoes and aubergines (egg plant), which are tropical plants. Although they may now be grown in temperate regions, they still retain their yin nature, as shown by their very high potassium and low sodium content. Among seeds and nuts, sesame, pumpkin and

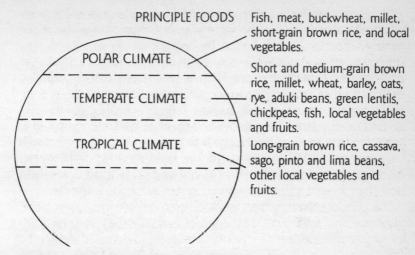

PRINCIPLE FOODS

POLAR CLIMATE — Fish, meat, buckwheat, millet, short-grain brown rice, and local vegetables.

TEMPERATE CLIMATE — Short and medium-grain brown rice, millet, wheat, barley, oats, rye, aduki beans, green lentils, chickpeas, fish, local vegetables and fruits.

TROPICAL CLIMATE — Long-grain brown rice, cassava, sago, pinto and lima beans, other local vegetables and fruits.

Figure 15. *Adapting diet to different climates.*

sunflower seeds, chestnuts, almonds, walnuts and hazelnuts are preferable to poppy seeds, Brazil and pistachio nuts. Fruits can be chosen from those growing in this country, such as apples, pears, strawberries and blackberries. Citrus fruits, dates, figs, pineapples and mangoes are generally not suitable. Food selection by this ecological principle is summarized in figure 15.

So it can now be seen that it is fine to eat oranges in Morocco, but apples and strawberries are better in Northern Europe or North America. A lot of fish and meat is necessary if you live with the Eskimos, but in our climate the body does not burn up all the animal fat, which accumulates in the body, causing numerous problems. However, if we travel to other parts of the World, we need to adapt ourselves to local conditions by eating the traditional diet of the locality. So a little wine can be enjoyed in Greece, a mild curry in India, and dates in Egypt!

FOOD FOR DIFFERENT SEASONS

People who live in a temperate climate experience quite big changes in weather throughout the year. They adapt naturally to these changes by eating more salads, fruits and cool drinks in the summer, and more hearty long-cooked soups and stews in the winter. As with adapting to hot and cold climates, we can maintain our health by becoming *more yin in the yang heat of summer, and more yang in the cold of winter*. Again, the easiest way to do this is to eat the foods that are available in our environment, as they change over the seasons.

In the spring and summer, there are plenty of greens, lettuces, radishes, peas, and green beans, and their cooling effect is ideal for the season. In the autumn and winter, kale, swedes, turnips, cabbages, and Brussels sprouts provide greater warmth. Some vegetables, like onions and carrots, grow and can be eaten through several seasons.

Among grains, the more balanced types like rice, wheat and barley can be eaten all year round. The more yang grains, such as buckwheat and

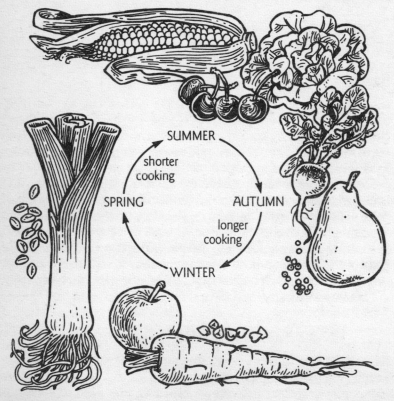

Figure 16. *Adapting diet to the changing seasons.*

millet, can be eaten more often in the winter to provide greater warmth, and the most yin grain, corn, can be eaten more often in the summer, giving more coolness.

In the summer, we can enjoy abundant fresh fruits. In winter, we can use the easily stored fruits like apples, as well as dried fruits like sultanas, raisins and apricots.

We can also eat more grains and less vegetables in the winter, and increase the amount of foods high in fat and protein, such as beans, seeds, oil and fish, to give more warmth. At this time, more longer-cooked recipes and a little more sea salt, miso and shoyu will also give more warmth and energy. In the summer, we can eat less grains and more vegetables, and use shorter cooking styles with less salt to retain the cooling qualities of foods. These seasonal adaptations are illustrated in figure 16.

FOOD FOR DIFFERENT INDIVIDUALS

As we pass through life we change a great deal, and our food requirements also change. Babies are small, compact and very active, or more *yang*. They therefore need a more *yin* diet for their normal upward growth and and development. In their first months their mother's milk is obviously ideal, its liquid form reflecting its more yin nature. At weaning, soft cooked grains, vegetables and other foods can be introduced, with very little salt. Until the age of 7 or 8, foods can be prepared with a gradually firmer consistency and with more salt. After this time, children can eat a normal adult diet. On reaching old age, people become slightly more contracted or yang again, and so need a little less salt and fish, and more lighter cooked foods. Further details on feeding babies and children are given in chapter 9.

Our past eating habits have formed our present state of health. Our overall condition may have become *too yang, too yin, or a combination of both*, as described in earlier chapters. In establishing our health, we can make adjustments within the Standard Diet to bring us back to a balanced condition. If you are too yang, you should eat less of the more yang foods like salt, fish and grains, and more of the yin foods like vegetables, fruits, pickles and alcohol. Among grains, buckwheat should be avoided, and a greater proportion of barley and corn eaten. Shorter and lighter cooking styles can be used more, and baked, burnt and overcooked foods should be avoided.

If you have become too yin, you should have less fruit, salad and alcohol, and more salt, miso, shoyu, fish and grains. Buckwheat and millet can be eaten regularly, as can well-cooked root vegetables, aduki beans and sea vegetables like kombu, kelp and hiziki.

If your condition is a combination of too yin and too yang, then both extremes should be minimized, with less fish and fruit. The more centrally balanced grains like millet, short grain rice and barley can be used most often. The use of salt should be moderate, and the most yang cooking methods like baking and the most yin like salads should be used infrequently.

Common sense tells us that people engaged in different activities have different dietary needs. More physical and social activities such as farming, labouring, public speaking, sports, and business management are more yang, and require a slightly more yang diet to sustain this activity. This can be achieved with more strongly cooked and seasoned food, and more protein and fat from beans, oil, seeds, nuts, and fish. More emotional, mental and spiritual activities such as art, writing, administration, office work, and religious or spiritual activities are more yin, and require a slightly more yin diet to promote these abilities. This can be achieved with lighter cooking styles, with little or no fish, and more of the yin varieties of grains and vegetables, such as barley, leafy greens and beansprouts.

Adapting your diet to different activities makes it easier to accomplish your chosen work and pursuits. Over a longer period of time, this knowledge also gives the freedom to choose those qualities and abilities that you want to develop in yourself. This can be a great aid in realizing your full potential, and taking the most constructive and enjoyable direction in your life.

Finally, we can look briefly at how dietary needs change at a very special time, during pregnancy. Extra care is needed to ensure that the additional nutritional demands of the foetus are met by the mother's diet. Larger quantities of foods rich in protein, iron, calcium and other nutrients are needed at this time. This can come from greater amounts of beans, bean products like tofu and tempeh, green leafy vegetables, seeds, and sea vegetables. Pregnant mothers frequently experience strong cravings for extreme foods outside the usual range of foods in the Standard Macrobiotic Diet. Efforts should be made to substitute the craved-for food with a similar but more healthy food, but if the craving persists it is probably wise to eat just enough to satisfy the desire.

During pregnancy, a great concentration of energy, blood and nutrients is creating the new life, which means that the mother becomes more yang. Therefore a more yin diet with less salt and lighter grain and vegetable dishes helps the mother to stay in good health and avoid some of the common problems experienced at this time. Further information on eating healthily during pregnancy can be found in the book, *Macrobiotic Pregnancy and Care of the Newborn Child*, details of which are given on page 156.

From this chapter we can appreciate the flexibility of the macrobiotic way of eating. It is important to realize that health is not a static state which, once reached, will continue indefinitely, but a continual act of keeping balance internally and with the environment. When beginning to eat macrobiotically, following the Standard Diet will have a strong effect in bringing you back into balance. Over time, you can then refine your cooking more and more for your personal needs, giving a continual improvement in health and emotional and mental well-being.

CHAPTER EIGHT

HOW TO BEGIN
EATING MACROBIOTICALLY

Here are twelve steps you can use to start on the macrobiotic way of eating. You may have taken some of these steps already, in which case you can begin further on. It is important to find your own pace in working through the steps. For some people, going too fast can lead to suddenly wanting to give the whole thing up. On the other hand, going too slowly will mean that the benefits of macrobiotic eating will take a long time to become apparent. You need to find the middle way which is right for you. Useful ideas on menu planning and recipes will be found in later chapters.

Step 1: Eat whole grains every day
Whole grains are the most balanced of foods, and you should eat them every day, and preferably at every meal. As explained before, these should be mainly whole grains with a smaller amount of flour products. You can start at breakfast by making a porridge with good-quality rolled oats (oats that come in cardboard boxes are usually pretty tasteless), or with rice, barley or wheat flakes. These are best cooked with water and a small pinch of sea salt, and can be seasoned with gomasio or roasted seeds, or sweetened with barley malt, rice syrup or apple juice.

For your main meal of the day, you can choose from a great variety of grain dishes. Short or medium-grain brown rice is very versatile, and can be cooked by itself or in combination with barley, wholewheat, millet, beans or chestnuts. After cooking, it can be mixed with roasted seeds or nuts, or mixed with vegetables to make a rice salad. Other grains like barley, millet and corn can also be used, and also various types of wholewheat noodles, pasta and spaghetti. Whole grains take a long time to cook, so it is a good idea to cook enough to last for several meals at a time.

For your other smaller meal, which may well be lunch away from home, it is easiest to take the grain and other dishes left over from your last main meal in a convenient container. Sometimes you could also make up a quick meal using sourdough bread, or noodles which are quick to cook.

Step 2: Stop eating eggs, meat and poultry

The second step is to *cut out the extreme yang foods*. If you are accustomed to using eggs, meat and poultry as the centre of meals, you will need to find new dishes to take their place. White fish and seafood are a good alternative. They can be cooked in many different ways, including frying, poaching, grilling, baking, and in combination with grains and vegetables. To create a better balance, they can be prepared with a yin seasoning like rice or cider vinegar, lemon juice, horseradish, mustard or grated root ginger. They should also be served with a generous helping of salad or greens.

Eventually, fish should form only a small part of your diet, and you should only eat them once or twice a week. As you get more used to the diet, grains and beans will take the place of animal foods, providing filling meals with a similar yang quality.

Step 3: Replace sugar with healthier desserts

Now we *cut out the major yin foods* in most people's diets. These include all forms of sugar and foods containing sugar, such as honey, molasses, commercially-made cakes, biscuits, chocolate, ice cream, sauces and many tinned foods. Check food labels before you buy foods.

To satisfy your sweet taste, learn to make better-quality desserts using fruits, natural sweeteners like barley malt, seeds, nuts and grains. These can be just as exciting and satisfying, and can include your own cakes and biscuits, fruit jellies, pies and crumbles, puddings and sweet sauces.

You may feel like having these every day at first, which is fine as they will be of a much better quality than bought desserts. In time, your need for them will lessen, and eating a dessert a few times a week will be sufficient.

Step 4: Learn to make soups

Home-made soups are incredibly delicious. Canned and packet soups bear no comparison to what you can make yourself quite simply. Vegetable soups can be quick to make, and are especially tasty if you use the water left over from boiling or steaming vegetables for other dishes. Seasoning with miso, tamari or shoyu will give a rich, full flavour to your soups.

This is a good time to begin using a little sea vegetable. A small amount of the quicker-cooking varieties like wakame or dulse can be chopped finely and cooked in almost any soup.

Step 5: Replace dairy foods with beans and bean products

Cutting out dairy foods is a difficult step for many people, but it is well worth the trouble. When they finally go, many people experience all kinds of benefits such as having clear sinuses for the first time in their life, less frequent colds and coughs, less ear problems and better hearing, and clearer thinking. Several foods can help with giving up dairy foods. Good-quality firm tofu resembles cheese in texture, and can be used in its place in many recipes. Seed and nut butters like tahini and sunflower spread can be used to replace butter and vegetable margarines, although they should eventually be used only occasionally because of their high oil content. Sugar-free soya milk can be used instead of cow's milk in some recipes, though in time this too should be used only occasionally as it lies at the yin end of the foods normally used in the Standard Diet.

As you reduce dairy foods, begin using beans regularly as a source of protein. They can be eaten every day, but should not form more than 5-10 per cent of your daily food—1-2 heaped tablespoons a day is sufficient for most people. Beans are far more digestible when cooked with a sea vegetable, so this is the second place you can introduce them into your diet. Suitable varieties include wakame, kombu and kelp.

Step 6: Stop using stimulants

These come in different forms, as beverages like tea, coffee, wine, spirits, aromatic herb teas and soft drinks, as seasoning like spices and herbs, cocoa, carob, ginseng, and sauces containing spices and chemical flavourings. In their place, use beverages like twig tea, grain or dandelion coffee, a moderate amount of apple juice, and traditionally-made beers such as Guinness. Start using seasonings like tamari, shoyu, miso, rice vinegar, grated root ginger, mustard and fresh parsley or chives. At first, you may miss the kick of strongly seasoned foods, but with time the sense of taste and smell generally becomes much better and the natural flavours of grains, beans, vegetables and other whole foods become very satisfying.

Step 7: Use foods produced in a temperate climate

This means cutting out tropical fruits like bananas, oranges and dates, and potatoes, tomatoes, aubergines (egg plants), and peppers. These all have a weakening effect on the body, and are easily replaced with the wide range of temperate fruits and vegetables growing in your locality.

If you have now accomplished all the above steps, well done! You are now approximately eating the Standard Macrobiotic Diet. Now you can take some further steps to increase the health benefits of your meals.

Step 8: Learn to plan balanced meals

Now that you are familiar with using the various foods in the Standard Macrobiotic diet, you can learn the art of creating balanced meals with them. Bear in mind two useful points. The Standard Diet plan shows *the proportions of different foods to eat in one day*, by volume on your plate. A meal could contain only one or two of the food types, as long as the other types are eaten at other meals on the same day to make up the correct proportions.

Secondly, because of the time it takes to prepare whole foods, it is a good idea to spend a reasonable time cooking the main meal of the day and make the others quickly-prepared meals. Also, if you cook more than you need for the main meal, some of the food can be used to make a smaller meal. This is particularly true for grains and beans which require longer cooking.

We can now look at how to plan the menus for the three main meals of the day, breakfast, lunch and supper.

Breakfast can be a simple meal of various types of porridge made with whole or rolled grains. Other possibilities are mashed tofu scrambled in a frying pan with tamari or shoyu and chopped spring onions or parsley; a light soup, or some noodles. Any left-over dishes could also be included.

Lunch can be made up of the dishes cooked at yesterday's main meal, a soup, or a quickly-prepared meal like noodles and steamed vegetables. If you eat lunch away from home, these can be taken in a plastic or ceramic food container, with soup or tea in a thermos flask.

On most days of the week, the main meal should contain a wide variety of dishes, including the following:

1. A soup, unless you have already had one that day.
2. A whole grain.
3. A variety of root, round and green vegetables. There should be a balance between some longer-cooked vegetables and some which are more lightly

cooked or eaten as pickles or salad.

4. A dish higher in protein, such as beans, tofu or fish.

You can also add the following several times a week:

5. Sea vegetables, such as arame, hiziki or wakame, cooked by themselves or with vegetables.

6. A dessert made with natural sweeteners, fruits and so on.

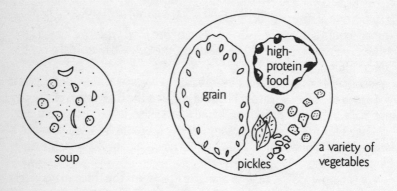

Figure 17. *Abalanced meal with a full variety of dishes.*

Your main meal may often look like that shown in figure 17. In this illustration, the different types of food are shown separately, but they could sometimes be combined—as a bean soup for example, or as a grain and vegetable stew. All this may seem to be a lot to prepare, but with practice you will find that it becomes second nature to cook meals with this variety.

Step 9: Reorganize your kitchen

You will already have done this to some extent, but some further reorganization will make your cooking easier and better. Start by thoroughly clearing out all the foods that you no longer use, and stock your kitchen with the macrobiotic quality foods you are now using. A great advantage of cooking macrobiotically is that most of the foods store well. This means that you can stock up once a week or once a fortnight, and only need to shop for fresh vegetables and fruit more frequently. With vegetables at hand, you can walk into the kitchen and cook a complete meal without prior planning. Figure 18 lists some of the foods that you may wish to keep a regular stock of.

Grains	Short or medium grain rice, barley, wheat, millet, rolled oats, wholewheat spaghetti and noodles, rice cakes
Beans and bean Products	Aduki Beans, green or brown lentils, chickpeas, kidney beans, split peas, tofu in the refrigerator
Sea vegetables	Wakami, kombu or kelp, arame, hiziki, nori, agar-agar
Seeds and nuts	Sesame, pumpkin and sunflower seeds, almonds, peanuts, chestnuts and walnuts
Dried fruits	Sultanas, raisins, pears, apricots, apple rings
Seasonings and condiments	Miso, shoyu, rice or cider vinegar, mustard, root ginger, gomasio, umeboshi plums, sesame oil, sesame spread
Natural sweeteners	Barley malt, rice syrup, concentrated apple juice
Beverages	Twig tea, grain coffee, apple juice, spring or well water

Figure 18. *Foods to stock up with.*

You may also need to get some new equipment for your kitchen. It is essential to have a good range of stainless steel, cast iron or enamelled saucepans and a frying pan or skillet. If you have aluminium or non-stick coated cookware, these should be replaced in time, because of their toxic effects. You also need a stainless steel pressure cooker for cooking grains and sometimes beans. If you have a wok, it will also come in useful for sautéing vegetables.

You will need a good sharp knife for preparing vegetables. A Chinese or Japanese-style knife made of carbon or stainless steel is especially easy and efficient for cutting and chopping. A brush with stiff bristles is also needed for scrubbing vegetables clean of soil and dirt.

Grains, beans, seeds, nuts, sea vegetables and other dried foods should be stored in glass jars or ceramic pots. These are preferable to plastic or metal containers which often affect the smell and taste of food.

Other useful items include a mesh strainer for washing grains, beans, and seeds, a grater for root ginger, a stainless steel or bamboo steamer, and a Japanese suribashi which is like a pestle and mortar but with fine grooves inside. It makes grinding seeds for gomasio very easy, and can also be used for puréeing sauces and dressings.

Most important of all is to keep your kitchen clean and orderly. This makes it a happier place where you can work easily and concentrate on producing appetizing and health-giving meals. In many ways, this is the most important room of the house, and the role of whoever cooks in it is the most important. In modern society the cook's work is often considered a lowly job, but in fact as the creator of health and emotional and mental well-being for all who eat his or her food, a good cook is not only valuable to families, but to the whole of society.

Step 10: Learn more variety

By now you will have learnt a basic number of recipes for preparing the different foods in the macrobiotic diet. Now it is time to branch out and learn a greater variety of dishes. Using the same few well-tried recipes all the time will lead to boredom, tiredness, and a desire for more extreme foods. Brown rice every day will kill almost anyone's appetite for grains! This is a time when people may give up eating macrobiotically, thinking that it is too limited and boring. However, it is not the diet that is limited, but the imagination and creativity of the cooking. *Variety is the spice of life* the old saying goes, and we need variety in our food to create variety in our lives. Variety in your cooking stimulates your appetite, and gives you vitality and a big appetite for life.

Cookery books are a useful source of recipes, and once you have mastered those in this book you can consult some of those listed on page 156. It can also be very helpful to attend some cooking classes, or share meals with other more experienced macrobiotic cooks. Once you have learnt the basic principles of creating balanced and healthful meals, you can also use your own imagination and creativity to produce endless variety in your meals. Some hints for creating more variety are given below.

Use a wide range of ingredients. There are at least a dozen different types of grains, beans and bean products, and fruits, many more types of vegetables, plus various additional foods. They can also be combined in many different ways to produce endless combinations.

Use a wide variety of cooking methods, such as boiling, steaming, pressure-cooking, baking, stir-frying and pickling. Carrots taste very different when baked, cooked in a stew, and grated in a salad.

Create different textures, such as dry and wet, crispy and mushy. A dry grain dish can be served with a sauce, and soft-cooked beans can be accompanied by crispy blanched salad or pickles.

Make use of the five basic tastes of food—sweet, sour, pungent, salty and bitter. The sweet taste is present in many foods such as some grains and beans, vegetables like onions and parsnips, fruits, and natural sweeteners. The sour taste can come from naturally fermented pickles, including sauerkraut, and rice or cider vinegar. The pungent taste is provided by spring onions, radishes, watercress, root ginger and mustard. A mildly salty taste can be given with seasonings like miso, shoyu and umeboshi, and from condiments like gomasio. The bitter taste is often present in kale and other greens, lettuce and celery. All or most of these tastes should be present in the main meal of the day, or at least eaten in the course of each day.

When a meal is balanced and contains plenty of variety, it will look appetizing and leave you feeling uplifted and fully satisfied. If you go looking for things to nibble at after a meal, it must have been lacking in some quality. Try to work out what quality was missing from the meal, and make sure you include it in the next. This is a great opportunity for learning to cook more balanced and appetizing meals.

Step 11: Dealing with cravings

Eating macrobiotically should not be a grim test of your willpower. Obviously, the more closely you follow the Standard Diet, the quicker the improvement in health, but unless you are trying to cure a specific illness, a more relaxed approach can be taken. You need to find the balance between eating as well as you can, and not becoming so strict that you build up a lot of tension and resentment.

Try to satisfy your cravings with the least harmful food you can, and don't feel *guilty* about it, as this can have a worse effect on your health than the food! Instead, enjoy the food, then enjoy getting back to macrobiotic eating.

A related problem is how to eat when you visit friends or family, or eat out socially. Dogmatically refusing to eat any non-macrobiotic food can create a lot of tension and resentment for you and other people. Generally, you can state that you do not want the most extreme foods like meat and sugar, while being more flexible in the range of other foods that you eat. Eating more widely occasionally is not going to be a big set-back for your health, as long as you are eating the best quality foods on a daily basis.

Step 12: Clarify your purpose

Eating macrobiotically often produces some new difficulties and challenges. If these are not to sway you from this way of eating, you must have a clear knowledge of why you want to eat this way.

We unconsciously use food to create different emotional and mental states in ourselves. A common example which everyone must have experienced is over-eating when faced with difficulties in order to deaden the senses and thinking. Other examples are eating a lot of yang foods to keep your emotions in, or eating more yin foods to keep up a spaced-out frame of mind. We can eat a lot of meat and salt to maintain an aggressive masculinity, or consume much milk and dairy food to keep a baby-like dependency and lack of self-sufficiency.

There is a strong force within each of us which makes us avoid change or growth, and stay in the same way of thinking and behaving. One method we use to do this is to *stick to the same fixed way of eating*. This vicious cycle is illustrated in figure 19. To break this cycle, we must change our ideas on what we want from life, like experiencing greater health and happiness, or greater emotional calm, or wanting to take more responsibility for our own health and life. A clear purpose gives you the motivation to continue with your macrobiotic eating.

Over months and years, learning more about macrobiotics and its practical application to your diet and health brings you to deeper levels of yourself. You reach a point where you don't need to worry about your physical health any more, and many unconstructive moods and attitudes like self-pity, anger, fear, frustration and depression diminish. At the same time, your true inner character and potentials are expressed more and

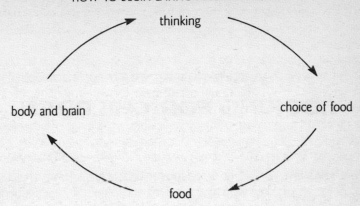

Figure 19.   *The cycle of choosing foods to create particular states of mind.*

more clearly. Sometimes we don't like these changes very much, and find that by eating more widely we can return to our old selves. Courage and willpower are then needed to continue on this path of self-discovery and change. However, this is the natural progress of life—continuous growth and change. It is the path to finding greater health, happiness and freedom in our lives.

CHAPTER NINE

COOKING FOR CHILDREN

If you have a baby or child, he or she too can benefit greatly from a healthier way of eating. Children who have been fed macrobiotically are frequently brighter, happier, more sensitive and receptive, and show less extreme behaviour like aggression and hyperactivity. As small children have a faster metabolic rate than adults, their condition changes more rapidly, and you often see a rapid improvement in their health.

Extra care is needed in looking after your children's health, as their rapid changes in condition can also mean that health problems come and go more rapidly. If your child develops any problems, it is well worth getting advice from other macrobiotic mothers or from a macrobiotic counsellor, and you should never hesitate in seeking the advice of a doctor or other health practitioner if you do not feel fully in control of the situation.

We have already looked at why dietary needs change with age. Now we can look in detail at the foods and cooking methods used for babies and children at different stages in their growth.

0-6 MONTHS

The ideal food for newborn babies is obviously their mother's milk. Scientific research now supports this view, showing that babies fed on formulas or cow's milk are more likely to develop digestive disorders or diarrhoea, have a lowered immunity to infections and illness, and have less chance of surviving the first years of life. In addition, some studies have shown that cow's milk can slow down the development of a child's intelligence, and skills like reading and spelling.

It is not difficult to understand why this should be so. At birth a calf's brain is almost 100 per cent developed, and in its first months of life its growth is mainly of the body—it often puts on 75lb (34kg) in the first six weeks. On the other hand, the human baby's brain is only about 23 per cent developed at birth. During the first few months, most of the baby's growth is concentrated on the brain, and he may put on less than 1 lb (450g) in the first six weeks. Appropriately, cow's milk is three times richer in protein than human milk and contains four times more calcium for the rapid growth of bones and muscles, whereas human milk contains nearly twice as much carbohydrate as cow's milk to nourish the growth of nerve and brain cells. Feeding calf food to human babies can increase their physical size more quickly, but at the expense of the development of their brain and intelligence. Breast-fed babies are generally brighter, more sensitive and alert than those fed on cow's milk.

While it is generally agreed that breast-feeding is preferable to artificial feeding for babies, many people begin feeding their children cow's milk after a few months. This will have all the effects described above, and also creates mucus in the lungs and associated lung problems, and in the ears causing common problems like ear-aches and partial deafness. It is often felt that cow's milk is necessary as a source of calcium, but many foods contain as much or more calcium, including greens like kale, broccoli and watercress, seeds and nuts like sunflower, sesame and almonds, and sea vegetables like dulse, agar-agar, kelp, kombu, arame, wakami, nori and hiziki. As long as children are fed the full variety of foods in the Standard Macrobiotic Diet, they will receive plenty of calcium. Parents should also make sure that their children spend a reasonable amount of time outdoors, so that their skin can make vitamin D which is necessary for the absorption of calcium from food.

While a baby is being breast-fed, his health will depend on that of his mother. The quality of a mother's food determines the quality of her blood, from which her milk is formed. Any changes in her diet will produce changes in her milk and the health of her baby. If a mother eats well, her baby will enjoy much better health and suffer less problems. When problems do arise, they can often be solved by making changes in the mother's eating. For example, nappy rash is caused by an excess of yin foods like sugar, fruits and spices, and will disappear if these foods are avoided. Ear-aches are often caused by the mother eating dairy foods or the yin foods just mentioned.

If a mother's eating is too yang, with an excess of salt, fish, and hard-baked flour products, the baby also becomes too yang. This often manifests itself as over-activity, with problems getting to sleep or waking in the night, screaming a lot, and wanting to feed excessively. If a mother's eating is too yin from fruits, fruit juices, desserts and so on, the baby becomes too yin. This often produces more docility and a lack of activity, a tendency to sleep a lot, and whining or whimpering rather than screaming. If the mother makes suitable changes in her eating, these kind of problems can rapidly improve.

6-8 MONTHS

At this time the teeth begin to appear, and babies often become interested in food, trying to put it into their mouths. This is the time to begin feeding them some solid foods. These must be specially prepared for them. Their needs are very different from the needs of adults, so they should not be given their parents' dishes. As they are more yang, they should not be given any salt or foods containing salt like miso, shoyu and umeboshi. Their food needs to be light and soft, so it should be cooked with more water and puréed with a suribashi, mouli, or baby food grinder. It should also generally have a sweet taste, similar to their mother's milk. Babies should not be given any buckwheat (the most yang grain) or ginger, mustard and horseradish, which are all too strong for their digestive system. You can begin to feed them the following foods.

1. Soft cooked grains
Soft cooked grains can form a baby's first solid food as it closely resembles their mother's milk. It is best to prepare your own with whole grains, rather than using grain flours or powders. Soya milk should not be used as its strong yin nature is very weakening for a baby's intestines and body as a whole. The most balanced and nutritious soft grain recipe is given below.

1. Take 4 parts short or medium-grain rice, 3 parts sweet rice, and 1 part pot or pearl barley. Wash the grains.
2. Put in a pot, add a 2-3 inch (5-8cm) piece of kombu or kelp sea vegetable, and 7-10 times as much water as grains.
3. Pressure cook for 1½-2 hours or boil for 2½-3 hours.
4. Purée in a suribashi, mouli or baby food grinder. At first, the consistency

should be the same as breast milk. This purée can be kept for 1-2 days, and used as needed. In hot weather keep it in a refrigerator.

5. Take one serving, add 1-2 teaspoons of barley malt or rice syrup to make the mixture the same sweetness as breast milk, and heat until just simmering.

6. Cool the purée and put into a baby bottle (you may need to enlarge the hole in the nipple a little), or feed with a small spoon.

From time to time, 5 per cent aduki beans or 5-10 per cent roasted and well-ground sesame seeds can be added to soft grain to provide more protein and oil. Cook the seeds along with the grains.

Sweet rice is used in this recipe as it is higher in protein than ordinary rice. If you have any problems getting it through your local food store, you can obtain it by mail order (see page 158).

When your child has been on soft cooked grains for a short time, the following foods can also be used on a daily basis.

2. Soups
These can be made from sweet vegetables boiled until soft. A small amount of sea vegetable like wakame, kombu or kelp can be cooked with the soup to add minerals, but these should be removed after cooking so that the child does not eat them. Soups should be puréed to form a drinkable liquid.

3. Vegetables
These can be lightly boiled or steamed and then puréed. Root, round and green leafy vegetables should all be used, especially sweet-tasting types like carrots, onions, swede, parsnips, white cabbage, cauliflower, leeks and broccoli. Greens can be tough and fibrous so they will need to be thoroughly puréed. If a baby does not find them attractive, they can be cooked with sweeter vegetables like onions and puréed together.

4. Sea vegetables
A small amount of sea vegetable can be cooked with grains, soups, and sometimes vegetables as a source of minerals. They do not need to be eaten, and can be removed from dishes after cooking. Care should be taken to remove all the salt encrusted on them before use—wipe them with a damp cloth or briefly rinse them in water.

5. Beverages
Once the baby has begun to eat solid foods, he or she will need some fluid

as well. You can use well or spring water, twig tea, roasted cereal teas like barley tea, and occasionally apple juice.

When your baby is regularly eating all these foods, there should be a balance of approximately 50 per cent grains to 50 per cent soups and vegetables.

8 MONTHS - 1 YEAR

During this period the number of breast feeds a baby receives can be decreased as the number of solid feeds are increased. Solid foods can gradually be made thicker by cooking them with less water. At first they should have the same consistency as breast milk, but by the age of 1 year they should have a more porridge-like consistency. A wider range of foods can be introduced, including the following.

1. Grains
Use a wider range of grains, such as 50 per cent short or medium-grain rice and 50 per cent barley, 75 per cent rice and 25 per cent whole oats, 75 per cent rice and 25 per cent sweet rice, and soft millet. Occasionally, a porridge can be made with rolled oats or rice, and wholewheat noodles can be introduced. These flour products are quite mucus-forming for babies, and should only be used a few times a week. Bread, dry crackers and pastry should not be given at all.

2. Beans and bean products
Beans, tofu and tempeh can be introduced on a regular basis. These are difficult for babies to digest unless they are properly cooked with other vegetables and a small amount of sea vegetable. They should be cooked until they are really soft all the way through to the centre. These beans and bean products can be mashed or puréed in the same way as other foods.

3. Seeds
Sesame, pumpkin and sunflower seeds can all be roasted, finely ground, and then sprinkled on grains and other dishes as a source of oil and minerals. It is better not to use nuts at this age, as they are difficult to digest and can cause digestive upsets.

4. Fruits
Fruits such as apples, pears, strawberries, and dried fruits like sultanas

and apricots, can be eaten several times a week. These should be lightly cooked and either mashed or puréed.

1-2 YEARS

Breast-feeding can be stopped four to six months after the first teeth appear, around the age of 1 year. The exact time will obviously vary a little from baby to baby. By the time a baby is weaned, he or she should be eating nearly all the foods in the Standard Macrobiotic Diet, in the correct proportions. Babies should be getting as wide a variety of ingredients and recipes as adults at this time.

Up until the age of 1 year, nearly all baby foods need to be separately prepared, but from this time onwards the baby can be given some adult dishes by removing a portion of soup, vegetables or beans before adding any salt or other seasonings. However, you will still need to cook grains separately, without salt. Not all foods need to be puréed. Some can be given in a more whole form as long as they are soft. Further variety can be added in the following ways.

1. Grains
Continue using a wide variety of different grains. These can sometimes be puréed, and sometimes eaten as whole, soft grains. Many children of this age enjoy corn on the cob.

2. Soups
At about 1½ years old, a very mild salty taste can be added to various foods, including soups, by using sea salt, miso and shoyu in *very* small amounts.

3. Vegetables
Use as wide a range of root, round and green leafy vegetables as possible. Children can manage large pieces now, and can be given cauliflower and broccoli florets, and squares of carrot, swede or parsnip.

4. Sea vegetables
When these are cooked with grains, soups, beans and vegetables they can be eaten along with the other foods.

5. Beans
A wide range of beans, tofu and tempeh can be used, cooked with a sea vegetable and either puréed or eaten soft.

6. Seeds and nuts

These can be used regularly, roasted and ground to a powder to make them more easily digested.

7. Fruit

Fruit can be eaten several times a week, usually cooked. It can be stewed, baked, or made into jellies using agar-agar flakes.

8. Fish

It is not usually necessary for small children to eat fish, but a very small quantity of white meat fish can be eaten occasionally. The fish should be cooked with vegetables to help create balance—for example, in a soup. Care must be taken as fish is a very yang food for small children.

9. Oil

A small amount of oil can be used three or four times a week, such as when stir-frying vegetables.

10. Grain sweeteners

It should not be necessary to use these to sweeten grains any more. Instead, they can be used to sweeten desserts like stewed fruit, jellies and rice pudding.

11. Seasonings

After the age of 1½, a little rice vinegar can be used, and light, non-salty pickles added to a child's diet.

2-6 YEARS

Over this period, foods can gradually be made firmer, so that by the age of 4, the child is eating food which is the same consistency as adult food. The amount of salt and salty seasonings can slowly be increased, and by the age of 6 or 7 children can eat the same dishes as adults, except for any especially salty dishes which should still be avoided.

Children have a natural attraction to sweet foods. This can be satisfied by making a wide range of good quality cookies, cakes and desserts. It will be much easier to feed children well if they have eaten macrobiotically from an early age. If you are just starting your children off on the macrobiotic way of eating, a certain amount of tolerance and broad-mindedness will be needed. If they feel they are being forced to eat this way, they may react by completely rejecting it. Parents may have to accept that their children will never eat as well as they would wish, and to some extent leave it up to their children to decide how they want to eat.

It is only possible to give a brief outline on feeding babies and children and how to deal with their health problems in this book. More information will be found in several books listed on page 156.

CHAPTER TEN

SOME OTHER SUGGESTIONS FOR HEALTHY LIVING

Eating a balanced and natural diet is fundamental to our health, but other aspects of our daily lifestyle are also important. In this chapter there are some suggestions for beneficial changes to your way of life that will give you greater health and energy.

1. *Eat only when you are hungry*. Our bodies tell us when we need food by giving us the sensation of hunger. Eating from habit or because it is meal or break time can lead to over-eating. Get in touch with your real appetite. Also, eat until you are satisfied but not overly full. Over-eating gives extra work to the body, and causes tiredness and a lack of appetite for other aspects of life. Two or three meals a day, with a few snacks if desired, are enough for most people.

2. *Drink only when you are thirsty*. The same applies as for food—your body tells when it needs more fluid by making you thirsty. If you are not thirsty, then you probably do not need any liquid. Some people advise a minimum daily requirement, such as 4 pints (2 litres). This is rarely necessary, and can over-work and weaken the kidneys. Have faith in your own body and what it tells you! When eating macrobiotically, a bowl of soup and between two and four cups of beverage a day are generally sufficient.

3. *Chew well*. We have been given teeth for a reason, so let's use them! Chew food until it is liquid before swallowing. This enhances the digestion of carbohydrates in the mouth by an enzyme in the saliva, and speeds the rest of digestion in the intestines. If you are eating whole natural foods, chewing well will also give you much more flavour and satisfaction from your food.

4. *Don't eat for three hours before going to bed*. Late-night snacks are

unhealthy for two reasons. Firstly, while you are asleep the body is working hard and gets no rest, so your sleep won't be as good and you will probably wake up feeling tired. Secondly, you cannot digest food properly when asleep, so it stagnates in the intestines and is improperly digested.

5. *Only eat when you are relaxed*. When you are tense or busy the digestive system is not prepared for food and does not digest it well. It is best to eat when you can sit down calmly and forget other matters. Having a brief silence, prayer or word of thanks before eating is a good habit to get into.

6. *Take regular exercise*. Our bodies are built to be used and regular exercise will keep them in good condition. We can get a lot of exercise from our daily routine, such as walking to work, cleaning the home, gardening, and so on. Some form of regular exercise programme, such as yoga, Do-in (self-massage), sports, or martial arts, is also very helpful. It is much more beneficial to take a moderate amount of exercise every day than occasionally attempt a bout of strenuous exercise.

7. *Use natural fabrics*. Clothes made of artificial fibres greatly reduce the natural flow of energy in the body and between the skin and the natural environment, especially when worn directly against the skin. Natural fibres like cotton, linen, silk and wool allow energy to flow, and are better for the health. Over time, it is also a good idea to replace artificial fibres in your home with natural materials. Bed sheets and pillow cases, towels, curtains, carpets and furniture coverings can all be changed. This can really change the way you feel in your home.

8. *Use natural cosmetics and toiletries*. Avoid using chemically-produced cosmetics, soaps and shampoos, as these can be damaging to the skin. Natural products made from vegetable sources are now widely available in health, wholefood and other shops.

9. *Use the minimum of electrical appliances*. Many modern conveniences, such as hair dryers, electric toothbrushes, shavers and blankets may not be good for the health. Scientific experiments have shown that most electrical appliances sap our energy when used close to the body for extended periods. They produce positive ions, which make us tired and tense. Various environments that are renowned for being peaceful, such as waterfalls, rivers and woods, produce the opposite, negative ions. Negative ions have a calming and energizing effect on us. If you have to use electric or electronic machines at work, it is particularly important

to create a more peaceful and healthy home environment. Having plenty of plants in your home or at work can be of great help.

10. *Don't take long hot baths or showers*. These can deplete your body of minerals and have a weakening effect. It is better to take fairly brief baths or showers, unless you have consumed a great deal of salt in the past. If you do feel weak after a bath, a cup of twig tea with a teaspoon of shoyu will help to replenish your energy.

11. *Dont spend too long watching television*. We take the television very much for granted, but long periods in front of it may not be good for the health. Colour sets, especially, have been known to emit low-level radiation, and spending a long time in front of them can be weakening. This is also true of computer display terminals and video games.

These suggestions are not hard-and-fast rules, but neither should they be taken too lightly. Reorientating our whole lifestyle with these points in mind is an important part of our overall development of health and happiness.

CHAPTER ELEVEN

THE MACROBIOTIC APPROACH TO SICKNESS

To know how to cure sickness, it is necessary to understand its cause. Removing the cause of the problem will then bring about a recovery. Unfortunately, the cause of most sicknesses is not generally understood in modern society. When most people become sick, they have no idea of why this has happened. Even a visit to a medical professional rarely ends with a clear explanation of the cause of a problem. If we do not understand the cause of a problem the only thing we can do is use a symptomatic treatment to remove the discomfort of sickness.

Because of this ignorance of the true cause of sickness, many people in modern society accept sickness as a natural, although undesirable, part of life. However, this need not be so. If we are prepared to find the real cause of sickness, we can enjoy our full lifespan in good health.

UNDERSTANDING SICKNESS

Most illnesses have four stages in their development. To help us understand these different levels of an illness, we can use the example of a very common problem, high blood pressure. You can work out the four levels of other illnesses quite simply yourself. The four levels are:

1. Symptoms
These are what we usually call sickness or disease, and include pain, stiffness, fever, vomiting, and coughing. In the case of high blood pressure, common symptoms include headaches, ringing in the ears, and giddiness.

2. Condition
The symptoms are produced by underlying conditions in the body, involving changes in blood quality, organs, nervous system and other

functions. With high blood pressure, the symptoms are caused by a rise in blood pressure. This usually occurs because of the constriction of small blood vessels, and sometimes also the enlargement of the heart.

3. Cause
The various abnormal conditions in the body have been caused by some aspect of a person's daily way of life. This can include diet, level of activity, living environment, and prevalent emotions. The principle cause of high blood pressure is a diet of extreme yin and yang foods, especially the over-use of salt. The yang foods cause the contraction of the blood vessels, and the yin foods cause expansion of the heart. As we saw in chapter 4, the cause of many illnesses is eating extreme yin foods, extreme yang foods, or a combination of the two.

4. Origin
Why does a person eat a diet that produces ill-health, not exercise his body, or maintain unhealthy emotions and general lifestyle habits? This must be because he or she lacks the understanding of how to live healthily. If a person develops high blood pressure, it is because he or she does not understand how to eat and live in a healthy way.

In society today there is a general confusion between the *symptoms* and *cause* of sickness. Generally, the symptoms of an illness, or the underlying condition in the body, are called the cause. However, they are not the cause at all, but just the result of the cause. For example, with high blood pressure it is well known that the underlying condition is the constriction of blood vessels and sometimes heart enlargement, and these are called the cause. But why have the blood vessels become constricted and the heart enlarged? The deeper origin and cause of these physical changes is a person's understanding of life, and how he or she puts this into practice in lifestyle and dietary habits.

Another example is our reaction to pain. Pain is thought to be the sickness, and we may try to eliminate it at all costs, never stopping to think about what the root cause of the pain may be. When we remove the pain we think that the sickness is gone, and that we are well again. But because pain is only a symptom and not the cause, we have not cured ourselves at all. We have just fooled ourselves into thinking we are cured. Sooner or later, the pain or other symptoms will return.

If we keep removing the symptoms of illnesses and ignoring their cause, we are really getting more and more deeply sick. Eventually we may develop some more serious sickness that makes us stop and think, 'How did this happen so suddenly?' If we had heeded the first signs of sickness, like pains, fatigue, or bad sleep, and improved our understanding of how to live healthily, we would never come to the crisis point that makes us ask this question.

Blaming illness on germs, bacteria or viruses is another way of confusing symptoms and causes. Many infections and other diseases are said to be caused by these micro-organisms, and it is thought that killing them will cure the disease. The real cause of these diseases is a weak body condition, that allows the micro-organisms to get into the body and flourish there. When an infectious illness like influenza spreads through a community, some people 'catch it' and other don't, because some people have a weakened and susceptible condition and other people's condition is stronger. It is also well known that many people carry the bacteria or viruses of tuberculosis, polio, AIDS, herpes and other illnesses, but do not contract the disease. Again, this is because their internal condition is just not suitable for the micro-organisms to grow and multiply.

Now that we have looked at the deep cause and origin of sickness, we can consider how to cure sickness at the deepest level.

UNDERSTANDING MEDICINE

Just as there are four stages in the development of any sickness, there are also four types of medicine, one for each level of sickness.

1. Symptomatic
Medicine at this level changes symptoms without treating the underlying condition or cause. Many drugs and medications fall into this level, including aspirin.

2. Conditional
Medicine at this level changes the condition in the body underlying the symptoms. This includes physical means like surgery, the use of many drugs, taking vitamin and mineral supplements, radiation therapy, and manipulative therapies correcting misaligned vertabrae in the spine and other distortions. It also includes some therapies that work on the flow

of energy in the body, such as acupuncture, shiatsu, homeopathy, and Bach flower remedies.

3. Causal
Medicine at this level changes various aspects of a person's way of life, including diet, level of activity, home and work environment and emotional experience. A wide range of therapists and individuals offer help at this level, from those giving detailed dietary recommendations or specific exercise programmes, to a friend giving a helpful word of advice.

4. Changing the origin
Medicine at this level is not what is usually called 'medicine', but is more like *education*. It offers people an understanding of why they became sick, so that they can heal themselves. This includes the macrobiotic study of the order of nature and the universe and its application to our health, as well as many other teachings. From these we can learn how to live our daily lives in harmony with nature's laws, in our diet, attitudes, relations with other people, and overall direction in life. This is the highest form of medicine, and it not only enables us to cure present illnesses at the deepest level, but also to secure health and happiness in the future.

These are some interesting differences between the upper and lower levels of medicine. Medicine at the first and second levels is very complex, recognizing many thousands of different diseases. You therefore have to study for many years to understand these forms of medicine. The third and fourth levels are simpler, ultimately recognizing only one sickness—a lack of understanding of life and how to live healthily. They are therefore within almost everybody's grasp, allowing people to care for their own health by changing their daily living patterns.

Symptomatic and conditional medicine views a patient in a fragmented way, looking at how to treat symptoms or parts of the body in isolation from the rest of the person. Its methods of treatment tend to be very artificial. Medicine for cause and origin takes a wholistic view of a person, including physical, emotional, mental and spiritual aspects, and offers guidance on reorientating that person's way of life towards a more natural way of living.

Symptomatic and conditional medicine also involves some other person doing something for you or to you, with very little change needed on your part. Medicine for cause and origin offers ways for you to take the responsibility for your illness, through making changes in your way of thinking and lifestyle.

This last difference has meant that the majority of people in modern society prefer to use symptomatic and conditional medicine as this is the easiest way out; you don't have to do anything about your illness yourself, but can leave it all up to the health professional. Over the last ten years this situation has been changing rapidly, with many people opting to use alternative therapies, and some choosing to make fundamental changes in their diet and lifestyle. There is also a small but growing number of people who are committed to the fourth level of medicine—learning about the order of the universe and its practical application, so that they can take complete responsibility for their health and lives. Life belongs to those who accept the responsibility for having it.

RECOVERY FROM SICKNESS

We experience health when we maintain a harmonious balance within ourselves, and between ourselves and our environment. When our daily way of life is out of balance, we become sick. At first the body attempts to restore balance through abnormal means, producing various minor symptoms. If these means are not enough to restore balance, we begin on a course of degeneration, which gives rise to more serious illness. Therefore all sicknesses can be divided into two types, *adjustment*, and *degenerative*.

Adjustment sicknesses usually come on suddenly, and are often short-lived, disappearing once balance is restored. They include the discharge of excess and toxins from extreme foods as mucus (which can lead to coughs and colds), some types of fever, diarrhoea, skin disease, headaches, migraines and some other pains, and emotions like irritability, depression, nervousness, or talking and laughing excessively. These minor illnesses are a warning that our lives are inharmonious, and that we need to make some changes in our lifestyle to avoid further illness.

Degenerative sicknesses most often come on gradually, slowly worsen, and do not disappear of their own accord. Sometimes the path of degeneration may go unnoticed, and then the sickness suddenly erupts as an acute problem. Some common degenerative illnesses are arthritis, rheumatism, heart disease and heart attacks, strokes, diabetes, cancer, asthma, hay fever, kidney and gall bladder stones, and long-standing moods and emotions like depression, worry, fearfulness, under-confidence, anger, and hypersensitivity. Mentally, this degeneration manifests itself in ways like stubbornness, prejudice, rigidity, scepticism, pessimism, and a general loss of direction.

Degenerative illnesses are cured by taking a path of regeneration and rejuvenation beginning at the fourth level of sickness and working up through the third and second to the first. Beginning at the fourth level means realizing that the origin of sickness is yourself. Through the choices you have made in life, you have set in motion the changes which end as sickness. This does not mean that you should feel guilty, for this has usually been done in ignorance. Feelings of guilt can incapacitate you so that you cannot make positive changes to recover your health. A more positive and constructive attitude to take is to realize that if we have caused the problem, then we can also solve it.

A change in thinking at the fourth level naturally leads to making changes at the third, improving our eating, activity, relations with other people, and general way of life. This in turn changes our internal condition, which can result in the symptoms disappearing.

This general course is effective with most sicknesses. However, if the degeneration has gone so far as to produce some serious or life-threatening problems, it may be necessary to supplement it with a more symptomatic approach for a limited time. This might be emergency surgery, a course of drugs, or some other therapy. At this time modern medicine can be very effective, and we should be very grateful for its help.

In using the macrobiotic approach to sickness, eating the Standard Diet and following the other suggestions for healthy living will clear up many minor health problems. With more serious and long-standing problems this approach will be made much more effective by getting detailed advice from a macrobiotic counsellor, and by attending classes in cooking and other aspects of macrobiotics.

CHAPTER TWELVE

SOCIAL AND GLOBAL IMPLICATIONS

Almost everyone today can see great problems in society and the world, and would like to see changes for the better. However, there is also a general bewilderment, and often despair, about how to understand these problems and how to solve them. To clearly understand their causes and possible practical solutions, we must take a broad view of our modern society. Beyond all other divisions based on economic, political, racial and social differences, there are two major currents in the world today.

The first current is produced by the microscopic, fragmentary and dualistic way of thinking that we looked at in chapter 2. This approach has tried to improve our health, happiness and quality of life with an analytical nutritional theory, symptomatic approaches to medicine, the greater and greater use of science and technology, and intensive farming methods, and has produced a separation of people into different groups with opposing views and objectives.

The second current is characterized by a more macroscopic or wholistic view of ourselves and the world. Examples include returning to a more natural way of eating and living, the use of wholistic approaches to medicine, movements working for the preservation of our natural environment, the use of more natural sources of energy such as sun and wind, the increasing popularity of organic farming and foods, concern for feeding the whole world, and many groups and organizations with the aim of developing people's wholeness, spirituality, and consciousness of the unity of all people on earth. This second current is rapidly gaining strength; even in the last decade the majority of people have become aware of this trend, and many have made changes in their diet, attitudes and lifestyle.

The first microscopic current has played a large part in creating many of today's pressing social and global problems. This includes the appallingly unhealthy modern diet and the decline in physical and mental health, the pollution and destruction of our environment through the thoughtless use of science and technology, farming methods that destroy the soil and at the same time the quality of foods and our health, a disintegration of social structure, the starvation of a large proportion of the world's population, and ever-increasing social and global conflict.

Most attempts to find solutions to these large-scale problems are still using the same microscopic and dualistic approach, including many political, economic, scientific and social ideas, and so are not providing effective answers. They often look for answers *out there*, in government policies, law and police systems, in the National Health Service, and in the increased used of science and technology. This approach tends to be symptomatic, attempting to change the outward symptoms of problems without considering their basic causes.

The answer to many problems lies in taking the more macroscopic view of the second current. The macrobiotic understanding has much to offer this current, with a new perspective on the problems in society and many practical ways of bringing about beneficial changes. Society is made up of individual people, and most problems in society originate at the individual level. Often problems are not *out there* but *in here* within each one of us, in a general loss of physical, mental and spiritual health and maturity. Solutions to larger problems therefore lie in the recovery of our individual health and view of life. A widespread change to the way of eating and living already described in this book would bring enormous benefits to society and the world. A further understanding of the macrobiotic approach to mental and spiritual health would bring about even greater changes in creating health, happiness and peace for everyone.

In this chapter we will look at some of the implications of the spread of the macrobiotic understanding on a number of aspects of society and the world.

RECOVERY OF PHYSICAL AND MENTAL HEALTH

At the present time, serious physical and mental illness is reaching epidemic proportions in modern societies. Despite great advances in medical research, more and more people are becoming ill. Many hospitals are full to capacity, with long waiting lists for some treatments, and the number of pills and medications taken runs into tens of millions. There is serious doubt about whether society can support the expense of such an enormous health-care system.

In the macrobiotic view, the size of our health-care system could be greatly reduced. At the moment, most people wait until they become ill before seeking medical help. If, instead, people learnt to prevent illness by making changes in their daily eating, living, and view of life, a much smaller health service would be needed. Eventually it could be a fraction of its present size, dealing mostly with the results of accidents and emergencies. Can you imagine living in a society where health is the norm, and serious sickness the exception? Well, it is perfectly possible. We have only to decide that this is what we really want, and to take the practical steps in our lives to bring it about.

HARMONIOUS SOCIAL RELATIONSI IPS

Every year there is a rise in the level of violent and socially destructive behaviour and crime in Britain and other modern societies. Common attempts to solve this problem have focused on increasing the punishment for various crimes, and strengthening the powers of the police and law. However, these are largely failing to reduce the problem. As with the modern approach to sickness, these approaches are trying to change the symptoms without addressing the cause, which is the declining physical and mental health of the individuals making up society.

The dramatic increase in social disorder should be of no surprise to us. Our physical, emotional, mental and spiritual aspects are part of one whole, so the well-documented decline in the physical health of society is bound to be accompanied by a decline in mental health, behaviour, and relations within society. It is probably no coincidence that the rapid rise in anti-social and criminal behaviour over the last few decades has coincided with the rapid decline in the quality of food and people's general eating habits.

The full recovery of physical health based on a more natural, macrobiotic way of eating is fundamental to solving this problem. Other attempts will be limited in their effectiveness unless this fundamental basis of behaviour is recognized. In understanding the connection between food

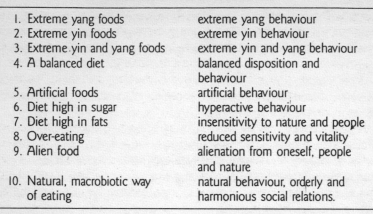

1. Extreme yang foods	extreme yang behaviour
2. Extreme yin foods	extreme yin behaviour
3. Extreme yin and yang foods	extreme yin and yang behaviour
4. A balanced diet	balanced disposition and behaviour
5. Artificial foods	artificial behaviour
6. Diet high in sugar	hyperactive behaviour
7. Diet high in fats	insensitivity to nature and people
8. Over-eating	reduced sensitivity and vitality
9. Alien food	alienation from oneself, people and nature
10. Natural, macrobiotic way of eating	natural behaviour, orderly and harmonious social relations.

Figure 20.   *The effects of different ways of eating on behaviour.*

and behaviour we can add six more principles to the four given in an earlier chapter. All ten are given in figure 20. We can look at the consequences of some of these principles on individual behaviour, life experience, and social relations in modern society.

Many people today are eating both *extreme yang and extreme yin foods.* This combination is especially likely to cause violent behaviour. Excessive yang food generates much tension and energy in the body, and with the extreme yin food this pent-up tension is often expressed explosively in abusive or violent behaviour. This combination can also create an abnormally strong sexual urge. Extreme yang foods like meat and salt stimulate the sexual energy in the body, and extreme yin foods like alcohol and sugar produce an urgent need for its release. This can result in aggressive and insensitive sexual relations, and is also a basic factor leading to acts of rape.

The majority of foods eaten today are *artificial.* Rather than being eaten in their whole, unadulterated form they have gone through various mechanical processes. Foods are broken up and disintegrated beyond recognition in refining, parts are thrown away—often the fibre, minerals and vitamins—and various chemicals are added to colour, flavour and preserve the food. Most of these foods would be quite unrecognizable as food by a person living one or two hundred years ago. The human species evolved over thousands of years, eating whole, locally available foods without chemicals. We have become adapted to digesting and metabolizing these naturally occurring foods. The typical modern diet produced in factories rather than fields, low in fibre, minerals and vitamins, and high in fats, simple sugars and chemicals, is going to produce a completely new and artificial condition in the body and mind. It should be of no surprise that physical and mental sickness and anti-social behaviour are so widespread.

A classic experiment carried out by a leading nutritionalist, Sir Robert McCarrison, demonstrated this very clearly. He was amazed at the health of the Hunza people living in the Himalayas, and concluded that this was due to their diet of primarily whole grains, with vegetables and a little fruit and dairy food. He fed this diet to a group of rats, who stayed healthy and raised healthy offspring, often behaving gently, playfully and affectionately. He fed another group of rats with a typical British diet of white bread, jam, sugar, tea and milk. This group soon acquired a host of physical diseases, and their behaviour was generally aggressive and vicious, including the eating of offspring. While we must be cautious in applying the results of animal experiments to our species, this study clearly shows the great effect an artificial diet may have in producing artificial behaviour.

The number one addiction in modern society is to *sugar*. From the first feed on manufactured baby foods, many people consume sugar on a daily basis. A high sugar diet has been shown to be a major cause of hyperactive behaviour. Sugar and foods containing sugar are well known to give energy, but it is absorbed into the blood stream so fast that the sugar level in the blood reaches abnormally high levels. This can give a person so much energy that he has to use it in some way or other, often explosively. Experiments in American Adolescent Detention Centres found that simply cutting all forms of sugar from the teenagers' diets brought about a drop in the number of violent incidents reported of between 45 and 80 per cent. The role of sugar in causing violent and criminal behaviour could be very high. These findings suggest that attempts to reform criminal and socially destructive behaviour should be based on a re-education of eating habits. This could have much greater long-term benefit than imprisonment for punishment, which has a high rate of repeated offences.

A typical modern diet contains plenty of *fat* in the form of eggs, dairy foods, meat, deep-fried and processed foods. As the body does not use all the fat, it is laid down in the body in and around the organs and under the skin. Fat is a great insulator of energy flow; it blocks the natural flow of energy within the body, contributing to physical health problems, and between a person and his natural and social environment. This reduces a person's sensitivity to his natural surroundings and to other people. It can contribute to an insensitive and egocentric way of relating to other people, with no concern for the health or welfare of others.

Over-eating has become a way of life for many people in modern society. However, eating more than the body needs makes extra work in digestion and in getting rid of the excess, and so reduces the energy available for other activities. This dulls thinking, vitality, and sensitivity and receptivity in relations with other people.

The typical modern diet is quite *alien* to our species. It is largely composed of foods that we could not naturally eat, including those imported from other climatic regions and grown out of season, factory processed foods, and chemical additives. This diet may be suitable for some alien race, but not for us! Eating an alien diet could mean that we will become aliens on our own planet.

Alienation means separation, and begins with a separation from our environment. Eating an alien diet, we lose our connection with nature and our adaptation to our natural surroundings. For example, if people living in a colder climate eat large quantities of tropical fruits and sugar in the winter, they feel cold. They then need to over-heat their home and work place to maintain a tropical environment as they have lost their adaptation to their local environment. This lack of adaptation leads to poor health and illness. When our foods are not taken directly from nature we also lose sight of the fact that we are composed of the same energy as our environment and are subject to the same order and rhythms that all nature follows. This can lead to a lack of order in all aspects of life, including behaviour and the way we relate to other people. One can believe that it is possible to do anything or be anything without receiving any unpleasant consequences.

Alienation from our natural environment creates alienation from ourselves. Our roots are in nature; every minute of every day we are fed and sustained by it. As our alienation from nature increases, so does our alienation from our own fundamental human nature and potentials. We then feel ungrounded, uncentred, and lose our sense of direction in life.

Everyone has unlimited potential for living creative and joyful lives, enjoying happy relations with their family, friends and community. Losing touch with this potential can bring about the feelings of worthlessness, hopelessness, fear and despair that are so characteristic of much of modern society.

Becoming alienated from ourselves leads to alienation from other people. In forgetting our own human potential, we forget that of others. This creates isolation, a feeling of separation from and often antagonism towards other people. With this view of the world it is easy to lose respect and concern for nature and other people, thus laying the way for anti-social and destructive actions.

As we have seen, the modern diet is a major cause of social disharmony, producing feelings of worthlessness, fear and despair, aggressive, violent and hyperactive behaviour, and insensitive, egocentric and alien relations between people. A return to a more natural, macrobiotic way of eating will greatly help the recovery of individual courage, optimism, and co-operation and sense of order in behaviour and relationships. This provides the fundamental basis of a more considerate and peaceful society.

CARE OF OUR NATURAL ENVIRONMENT

Mankind has left his mark on every corner of the globe. Everywhere there are signs of the pollution produced by Man's activities—in the soil, air and oceans. Enormous areas of the earth's surface have been completely changed or destroyed. This pollution and destruction is the result of a microscopic and dualistic attitude to nature. Nature is seen as quite separate from ourselves, and often as an enemy to be waged war with, conquered, and pillaged. This attitude also often fails to see beyond the present moment, ignoring the effects that our present actions will have in the future. 'Anything goes', as long as it satisfies immediate needs and desires.

A macroscopic view of ourselves on this planet gives a very different picture. We are one with nature. The sun, air, water, soil and plants have created us and continue to nurture us, so any changes in these elements and life forms will produce changes in us. Our health is completely dependent on the health of our whole planetary environment. If we wage war on nature, we make war on ourselves, pillaging nature means that we pillage our own bodies; as we pollute our environment we pollute ourselves, as we destroy the health of soil, we destroy the quality of foods and then our own health.

There are many similarities between our relationship with the planet and that of a cancer in the body. Like a cancer, we have become separated from the rest of planetary life; we no longer serve the healthy functioning of the whole but only our own ends, we draw on the general supply of resources but contribute nothing in return, and replicate endlessly at the expense of the whole. This cancerous relationship between mankind and nature on a large scale can be seen as the most basic cause of the small-scale development of cancer within us.

When we fully realize the unity of humanity and nature, the care of our natural environment becomes as important as the care of our own health. Individually and collectively, the preservation of our natural environment should be a top priority. In this we can learn much from many so-called primitive cultures who experience a deep connection with nature. They have a deep respect for Mother Earth, taking no more from her than is needed, removing only that which she can replenish, always considering the future effects of their actions for generations to come. Adopting this relationship with nature does not mean that we have to give up the idea of technological development, but that if we are to be free to enjoy its benefits, it must be carried out in harmony with nature. Technologies and manufacturing methods must be found that do not harm or deplete the environment, now or in the future. This should present no great problem for human ingenuity. It merely needs a reorientation in values based on seeing that we and our environment are one. As much consideration should be given for the health of the natural environment as we give ourselves, for in the end, both are the same.

REJUVENATION OF AGRICULTURE

The way in which our food is grown is not generally regarded as an important social issue, but in fact it has a tremendous effect on the physical, mental and spiritual health of society. Our food is our most intimate connection with nature. We take plants and animals from the fields and seas, and bring them within us into our digestive system where they are transformed into our blood and body. The primary concern of modern agriculture is economic—how to produce the greatest quantity of food for the least amount of money. The most important aspect of growing food, to sustain and optimize our health, has largely been forgotten. A change in values is needed, from producing the largest *quantity* to growing the best *quality*.

Many modern grains, vegetables and fruits bear little resemblance to their ancestors that have sustained our evolution over thousands of years. The breeding of new strains of crops and the use of chemical fertilizers has made foods larger, but with less flavour and vitality. They have a higher water content and contain less minerals and vitamins. Eating these devitalized foods makes us physically, mentally and spiritually weaker.

The last five years has seen the rapid spread of the organic growing of foods, without chemical fertilizers, herbicides and pesticides. This is a great step in the right direction, but our foods could be made still more vital by using the principles of natural agriculture. This system was pioneered by Masanobu Fukuoka, who has written several books on the subject from over three decades of experience (these are listed on page 156). Fukuoka realized that nature provides all our needs, and the closer we can get to allowing nature to grow our foods with the minimum of human interference, the better the quality of the food. His methods are easier to put into practice on a small scale, so if you grow any of your own food in a garden or allotment you can experiment with them yourself. The four most basic principles of natural agriculture are given below.

1. Non-weeding
Weeds occur naturally with food plants, and increase the fertility of soil through the tilling action of their roots and the micro-organisms that thrive among their roots. Some varieties, such as clover, also replenish the soil with nitrogen. When beginning, it might be necessary to replace larger weeds with smaller more desirable kinds.

2. Non-ploughing
Fields are ploughed to till, or turn over the soil, bringing nutrients up to the surface for crops to feed on. However, when weeds and organisms like earthworms are allowed to remain, soil is naturally turned over, making ploughing unnecessary. Furthermore, naturally tilled soil keeps a crumb-like structure that drains easily yet at the same time retains water for plants within the crumbs. Ploughing destroys this crumb structure, leading to problems with poor drainage, and drying out at the surface. Dry topsoils

are also prone to being blown away, which has caused great problems for modern farms in many parts of the world.

3. Non-fertilizing
Modern agriculture destroys all plants other than the crop species, and removes most or all of the crop once it has ripened. Not surprizingly, the soil becomes depleted in nutrients, requiring artificial fertilizers to keep up yields. If weeds are left, they naturally replenish the soil when they die. Returning the unused portion of crops further helps to maintain the soil's fertility.

4. Non-spraying
The need to use chemicals to kill pests has largely come about because only a single plant species is grown over a large area. Any insect pest entering a whole field of its favourite food plant is almost bound to multiply rapidly and cause extensive damage. We have inadvertently created paradise for these insects! It is the unnatural situation of large areas of one plant, found practically nowhere else in nature, that causes pest problems, not the insects. If land is kept covered by weeds, and different food plants are planted together—such as a root crop with a leafy vegetable—the problem of pests is minimized. The traditional practice of crop rotation, growing different crops in a field from year to year, also helps as the pests of one food species left in the soil rarely attack the different species grown the next year.

These principles may seem impractical to our modern way of thinking, but they have been shown to be quite workable. One might also think that these methods would give lower yields of crops, but Fukuoka has shown that he can get yields as good as or better than his neighbours who are using modern farming methods.

FEEDING THE WORLD

Faced with the problem of starvation on a huge scale, many modern efforts have focused on growing more food by developing new strains of crops, increasing the mechanization of farming, and using chemical fertilizers and sprays. However, these have largely failed to produce the food needed by the third world countries containing the majority of starving people.

Taking a broader view, the simple fact is that there is *already more than enough food* grown in the world today to feed everyone adequately. Enough grain is produced to provide every person with more than 3000 calories a day, and then there are beans, vegetables, fruits and other crops. The apparent shortage of food is created by the unequal distribution of what is already grown, especially between the more technologically advanced countries and the third world. This is mainly due to the choice of diet that people in the USA, Britain, and other developed countries make, with large amounts of meat and dairy foods. It takes 8-10 lb (3½-4½ kg) of grain or other plant food to produce 1 lb (½ kg) of meat. So choosing a diet based on animal foods means that one consumes far more of the world's food supply than a non-animal food eater.

About one half of all the grain produced in the world is fed to animals to satisfy the demand for meat and dairy foods. It has been estimated that if instead this was eaten directly by people, there would be enough food to feed one and a quarter times the present world population. A clear example of how this leads to starvation can be seen on a smaller scale by looking at just one country, Mexico. Here, more than half of the grain grown is fed to livestock, which is mainly exported to the USA to be made into hamburgers, while 80 per cent of children in rural areas are under-nourished.

It may seem that we are personally incapable of taking effective action to feed the starving of the world, but we can, immediately, by changing the foods we choose to eat. A basic feature of the macrobiotic way of eating is its economy. Based on whole grains, beans and vegetables, it contains everything that we need for our health, and little more. With it, we can use the smallest share of the world's food supply, enabling everyone on our planet to eat adequately for their health.

SOCIAL AND GLOBAL HARMONY

Every level of the modern world is characterized by conflict. Most people are worried about the threat of total annihilation of humanity through nuclear warfare. Whether this occurs or not, the present world contains many wars, and at a social level there are many conflicts between various groups based on religious, political, and ideological differences. At the personal level, there is increasing conflict and division within families and between individuals. Conflict and the 'fight for survival' lie at the base of modern society and many people's everyday experience. Yet almost everywhere we also find the dream of *one peaceful world*. Why is it that we seem incapable of realizing this universal dream?

The root cause of large-scale conflict must lie in the way of life of the people making up societies. The problem is not so much *out there* with other people as *in here* within our own attitudes and behaviour, so attempts to produce large-scale changes must be accompanied by self-change. A microscopic and dualistic way of thinking naturally leads to conflict as we see ourselves as separate to other people, and nations as separate to each other. If we are quite separate, then it seems that we have something to gain from winning a conflict, and war becomes a viable way of life for securing personal needs and happiness. However, this separation is an illusion. Just as individual cells make up the body, we make up humanity. As the health of a cell depends on the health of the body and the health of the body on the health of its cells, our health and happiness depends on that of humanity as a whole, and the health of humanity depends on each of us.

In our personal efforts to create global peace we can change ourselves physically, psychologically and spiritually. At the physical level, separation and conflict exists in our cells and body. Physical imbalances and rigidity mean that we are out of step with nature, we have separated ourselves from it and from other people. Through eating macrobiotically in harmony with the order of nature, this separation slowly disappears. As we have seen in previous chapters, regaining our physical health and balance dissolves many illusions in our emotions and attitudes that lead to conflict, such as fear and insecurity, suspicion and mistrust, intolerance and aggression. A return to a natural way of eating and cellular health is a fundamental step towards creating social and global peace.

Psychologically, we need to remove the many artificial ways of separating ourselves from other people—for example, with the idea of nations. When we look at a map we see lines dividing up the land and sea into countries, but if we sail over the sea or walk across the land we will not be able to find them. National boundaries do not exist in nature, they are figments of our imagination that hide the unity of all mankind. In all areas of life, we can remove these barriers with a firm resolve to understand other people's views and ideas, and overcome all differences of nationality and race, tradition and culture, belief and ideology.

The spiritual realization of our unity dissolves the need for conflict. If you have an argument with another person and he 'wins', you are unhappy; if it ends in your 'winning', he is unhappy, and that unhappiness affects you. There is no way that you can win an argument or conflict; the only way you can create a gain for yourself is by creating a gain for the whole of humanity.

When we reorientate our personal lives in a peaceful and harmonious way, this will spread outwards to our family and friends, to our community and society, and to the whole of humanity. Every minute of the day, we are personally creating our society and global consciousness, and every minute we can add to the overall peace and happiness through our own health, thoughts and actions.

IN CONCLUSION

To bring about the changes discussed in this chapter requires all of us to think deeply about the basic philosophy of life which underlies modern civilization and many of our own personal views. We must turn from the exclusive use of microscopic and dualictic ways of thinking to include the macroscopic and wholistic way, based on an understanding of the order of nature and the universe. This requires a change from the present man-can-do-better attitude, to gratitude for what nature provides for us and humbleness for what it can teach us. Further, it requires our personal acceptance of responsibility for creating these various social problems through our own thoughts and actions, and a positive commitment to make changes in our personal lives that will create the changes we desire in society.

Of all the problems facing us, the degeneration of health is perhaps the greatest and most important to change as it lies at the base of many other problems. Our ability to make clear mental judgements and create harmonious relationships rests on having good health. When we lose our physical and mental health we can no longer contribute to the creation of a healthy society. Establishing our health is the basis of developing our happiness and social maturity, so that we can give help to our family, friends and community, and contribute to forming a happy, peaceful and harmonious world community.

CHAPTER THIRTEEN

THE MACROBIOTIC WAY TO HAPPINESS

Macrobiotics is not limited to food and health, but also offers a way to realize our full potential for happiness; it enables us to live life as an art, creating the life that we want. Nearly everyone wants to be happy, yet often do not know how to go about creating this. George Ohsawa's teachings on the order of the universe can help in showing how we can all do this for ourselves.

THE SPIRAL OF CREATION

The essence of Ohsawa's reinterpretation of worldwide ancient wisdom is his spiralic view of the creation of the universe and our world. A similar description can be found in the first book of the Bible, Genesis, in the ancient Taoist book, the Tao Te Ching, and in other ancient writings. In his interpretation he saw that creation occurred in seven stages, with human beings as the final product, as shown in figure 21.

The idea of One Infinity, God, or a state of absolute oneness is universal and is given different names by different cultures. Likewise, it is universally recognized that One Infinity divides into two opposite tendencies, or yin and yang, which create the material world of energy, matter, plants and animals. Everything in the material world is created by yin and yang, and so are relative to one another, unlike One Infinity which is undivided and absolute.

The beginning of the material world is energy, in the form of electromagnetic waves such as light, X-rays, and radio waves. On earth, we are bathed in a sea of waves coming from the sun, moon, planets, stars and outer space. The collision of different forms of energy form pre-atomic particles like electrons and protons. Modern physics has shown

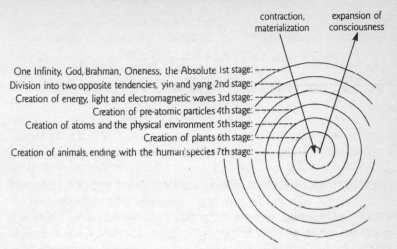

contraction,
materialization

expansion of
consciousness

One Infinity, God, Brahman, Oneness, the Absolute 1st stage:
Division into two opposite tendencies, yin and yang 2nd stage:
Creation of energy, light and electromagnetic waves 3rd stage:
Creation of pre-atomic particles 4th stage:
Creation of atoms and the physical environment 5th stage:
Creation of plants 6th stage:
Creation of animals, ending with the human species 7th stage:

Figure 21 *The spiral of creation and path of spiritualization.*

that energy changes into matter and back again in this way. Pre-atomic particles combine to form atoms, in a variety of elements like hydrogen, oxygen and carbon. Atoms combine to make molecules like carbon dioxide and water. Atoms and molecules form our physical environment, the air, water, rock and soil.

Plants are formed by the elements. They take up air, and water and nutrients from the soil, and use the energy of sunlight to create organic molecules and cells. Plants are eaten and become animals, which have evolved from simple one-celled organisms to the most complex, the human species. So we can trace our origin back through the other levels, and find that plants are our parents, the elements our grandparents, and so on back to our origin in One Infinity.

The spiral of creation is a yang process of contraction and materialization. This yang process must be balanced by a yin process. This is the expansion of our human consciousness back to One Infinity. Just as our origin in One Infinity is universally recognized, so is our destiny to return to it through our development of consciousness and spiritual growth. This is the aim of religions and many philosophies world wide. As the yang spiral ends with our species, we are the most yang of all forms and have the greatest capacity for the yin expansion of consciousness.

THE PATH OF SPIRITUAL DEVELOPMENT

The process of creation can be divided at the third stage into the higher stages which are more subtle (yin) and the lower stages which are more gross or material (yang). Western science is restricted to studying the more gross levels of creation, because it relies on using our five senses to observe the world. The more subtle stages can be studied using the intuition or 'sixth sense'. When our awareness is in the lower material stages it seems that we are all distinct and separate entities. This gives the illusion of 'I', the small self, or ego. As an awareness of the more subtle stages develops, this separation dissolves and we feel part of a greater whole, of humanity, the world, and eventually the whole universe. This means living from the big Self, having universal awareness, and consciousness of One Infinity. We are all somewhere on this path, from living for the self to realizing that we are the Self.

All difficulties and unhappiness come from living from the small self and identifying ourselves with the ego. As consciousness rises to more subtle and larger spheres, conflicts and unhappiness disappear. An example of this is anger. As we have seen, our physical condition can make us more angry, especially if we become too yang. Another cause of anger is living from the small self, where we think of ourselves as being separate from other people, objects and events. The very essence of anger is that we are angry at *someone or something else*. But when we realize that they or it are actually a part of us, there is no possibility of anger, there is no 'other' to be angry at! When we watch an angry person from a detached point of view, he can seem very funny—how can he take himself so seriously? If we can take this objective view of ourselves, our anger will also seem amusing! It will then evaporate, often into laughter.

Another example is fear. Again, our bodily condition can make us more fearful, especially if we have become too yin, but there is also a psychological and spiritual cause. When we cling to our small view of the world and to the self, we can fear that other people or forces will take away our money, possessions, friends, or our life. If we experience difficulties, conflicts or illness, we fear losing or dying. Viewed from the large Self, it is only our small self that loses or dies, the Self lives on, for the self is short-lived and the Self is eternal. Realizing that we are the Self means that we cannot lose anything, we have everything already, and there is no cause for fear.

The level of our happiness depends on how far we have grown from our small, egocentric view of ourselves towards realizing our unity with our family, friends, all other people, and the natural world. When you encounter any difficulty you can try this out. The fact that you experience difficulty means that you are living from your small self. Take a broader view that encompasses the source of the difficulty—another person, situation or event—and the difficulty either dissolves away, or you realize how to solve it in a harmonious and constructive way. Either way, you don't have to be unhappy!

PRACTICAL STEPS TOWARDS HAPPINESS

We are all living in the material and subtle worlds. Becoming over engrossed in either the yang material world or the yin subtle world can bring unhappiness from the other aspect that is ignored. Many people live for only one or other of these aspects, and so limit their happiness. Many thinkers and philosophers only teach about one or other aspect, and so limit the happiness that their teachings can give to others. For our happiness, we need to pay attention to both aspects. They are the *yin and yang sides of life*. The spirals of creation and spiritualization reveal some practical steps for developing our happiness in our material and spiritual lives, some of which are given below.

1. Use macrobiotic principles in your eating
Our ability to move on the outward path of spiritual development depends on the quality of our bodies and minds formed by what we take in from the incoming spiral of materialization. This includes our plant and animal food, water, air, light, and other forms of energy such as ideas and insights. If we want to develop our consciousness to more subtle levels, we must take in more subtle food and less material food. This means that plant foods are preferable to animal foods (traditionally, this is almost universally recognized by religions around the world), and that we should take less plant food and more mental and spiritual food.

The macrobiotic way of eating produces a quality of the body and brain for the fastest development of consciousness. It is based on the highest principle possible, creating oneness inside us through the harmony of yin and yang in our food. There is a tremendous force, the Will of One Infinity, moving us outwards on the path of spiritual development. We have to really get in the way to prevent this movement. One of the main ways that many people block this natural flow is through choosing foods that reduce their physical, mental and spiritual vitality, and block the flow of energy through their body and brain. The simplest thing we can do to make this path easy is to make our body and nervous system a clear channel for this natural flow.

2. Develop your understanding of the order of the universe
Everything in the relative world is formed by and changes according to the order of the universe—the spiral of creation and spiritualization, and yin and yang. In this book we have looked at this order in food, health and sickness, behaviour and social problems. We can also see that all other aspects of nature and our lives follow this order.

We spend most of our time using our sensory, emotional and intellectual consciousness. We often think we want this and not that, this is pleasurable and this is unpleasurable, this is beautiful and this is ugly, this is wrong and this is right. All these divisions are only relative judgements, and keep us in the relative world. When we can take a detached point of view and see that everything happens in an orderly way according to the unchanging order of the universe, we raise our consciousness from this small world to appreciate the greater whole. From this viewpoint we can see past our small everyday experiences to the greater order and harmony of nature. Then nothing seems inharmonious, and there is no cause for unhappiness. Everything happens in perfect order.

3. Develop self-responsibility
We are the creators of our lives. Only we can improve our happiness and quality of life. If we suffer from sickness, poverty or unhappiness, it is we who have caused it. Through our ignorance of the laws of nature, in our eating, conduct and behaviour, we have brought these on ourselves. We can change these to health, richness and happiness through our own thinking and actions. No one else can do this for us, we must take the initiative to change for ourselves. Of course, we can get advice and guidance from others, but ultimately it is only we ourselves that can bring about changes.

This can be a difficult lesson to learn in modern society because the educational system largely creates dependency, rather than teaching people how to care for their own health and take the initiative in deciding how to lead their lives. Once we reach maturity, blaming other people or events for problems is no longer a valid excuse for our difficulties, and we can realize the possibility of fully directing our lives. With a growing understanding of how all events and changes in our lives follow an orderly pattern, we can become masters of our destiny, creating health, happiness and freedom. With this understanding of the forces of nature, one's experience of life changes from that of a *victim* to that of a *player of life's game*. We can choose the challenges and games that we want to produce our happiness and further development.

4. Be grateful for difficulties

Modern society is becoming increasingly intolerant and fearful of difficulties. Many technological devices are thought to be essential to make life more comfortable, and many methods of escaping from everyday reality are popular. This fear is a result of a lack of health, vitality and vision to cope with difficulties and create a better situation. When we regain our health and vision, difficulties can be embraced as positive stimuli for our growth, allowing us to find our limitations and grow beyond them. They are our greatest teachers! If we live without challenges, we tend to stagnate and stop developing, and life becomes monotonous.

When we climb a mountain or set out to accomplish a plan, the more hardship we experience, the greater the joy on reaching the top of the mountain or putting the plan into action. The more seriously sick we become, the more we appreciate health. Avoiding difficulties is really the cause of unhappiness, and meeting and growing beyond them is the cause of happiness. In order to develop greater happiness, we can continue to give ourselves difficulties.

5. Use the front and back law

In the relative world everything is formed by both yin and yang in varying proportions. Therefore everything has two sides to it, the front and the back. This law helps us to understand many things in our lives, for anything which on the surface seems to be a great advantage for us also carries some deeper disadvantage with it. Thus modern industry makes our lives more comfortable and easy (the front), but at the same time poisons our natural environment, food and health (the back). If we become rich (the front), it is because others are poor (the back). Also if we become rich in material possessions (the front), it is often because we have ignored and become poorer in our spiritual awareness (the back). We may enjoy a few minutes pleasure from eating an ice cream (the front), but the next day our health suffers and we may experience discomfort (the back).

This law can also be seen the other way around. The rising tide of degenerative illness (the front) has led to great interest in returning to a more natural and healthy way of living and eating (the back). The present threat of the greatest human destruction by nuclear warfare (the front) has led to a strong movement for peace (the back). When we realize that we have acted selfishly and small-mindedly (the front), we become more humble and considerate (the back).

There is a natural harmony or balance between yin and yang, or front and back, so the bigger the front, the bigger the back. For example, modern drugs can bring the quickest and easiest relief, but their damaging side-effects are often the greatest. Money brings comfort and joy, but some of the richest people in the world are also the saddest. Rising to a position of great power or status attracts the most enemies, and is followed by the greatest fall. The nuclear bomb is the deadliest weapon ever created, giving great power, but if the enemy also has it, it makes one very weak.

It is interesting to see that modern society has gone for creating the biggest front possible in many aspects of life, and consequently also suffers the biggest back. Clearly, the front and back law is not widely understood! When it is, society can avoid many of its present problems and become much healthier and happier.

We can individually increase our happiness by living more humbly and modestly; if we do not create a big front, we will not experience a big back. By taking only what we need in material goods, we do not later become materially or spiritually poor. Rather than making ourselves the first or highest in position or status, we make ourselves the last or lowest, then we will receive far more from other people and the universe. If we do rise in position, we can avoid the back by becoming more humble and serving more people. If we humbly give respect and love to other people rather than 'blowing our own trumpet', we will receive the respect and love of others. The greater our humbleness, the more we will receive.

When we experience difficulties or low points in our lives, there must also be a front to the situation. Often this is a time when we can learn the most. If we reflect on our difficulties and keep our optimism, we can reap the benefits of the front of the situation.

6. Develop gratitude

We often only look at all the things that we would like but do not have in life, which makes us unhappy. Actually, we receive so much—food, air, water, friends, children, and life itself. If we develop a deep gratitude for all that we receive, we can become very happy. Every day, every hour and minute we can feel this gratitude for things large and small. Try it—it can change your life!

7. Live the spirit of one grain, ten thousand grains

This is a very ancient Eastern saying, which reflects a general law of nature. Planting one seed produces many seeds, and when these are planted they produce thousands of seeds. Nature is endlessly multiplying itself. The path of our spiritualization is also one of expansion, and living by this law of nature will speed our progress. We can do this by endlessly giving; anything we receive we can give out many times over. When we eat, we can give out the energy from it to help many other people. If we are given love, we can return this to many people. If we learn something valuable, we can tell many other people about it.

Doing this will make many people happy. You will then receive this happiness back. The more one gives, the more one receives, becoming lighter, brighter and much happier.

CHAPTER FOURTEEN

MENU PLANS

This chapter gives menu plans for two full weeks' meals. With these you can learn how to create balance in your cooking, in individual meals, over one day, and with the seasons. Recipes for all the dishes are given in the next chapter.

The plans are designed to show the wide variety of possible dishes which can be served at different meals. You may find that certain dishes suit your appetite and lifestyle better. For example, breakfast can include a soup, various types of porridge with gomasio, roasted seeds or barley malt, scrambled tofu, lightly cooked vegetables, or pickles. Lunch can be made up of some of the dishes from yesterday's main meal or it can be a freshly prepared meal. Supper usually includes a soup if one has not been eaten earlier that day, a grain, a bean, tofu, tempeh or fish dish, a variety of vegetables, and sometimes a seaweed dish, but within this basic plan there are many ways of preparing each of these types of food. So try using these menus, and see which suit you best.

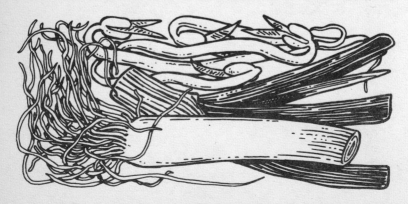

SUMMER MENUS

BREAKFAST

Monday

- Soft rice.
- Steamed spring cabbage.

Tuesday

- Rolled oat porridge.
- Boiled broccoli.

LUNCH

- Wholewheat or udon noodles.
- Onion, broccoli and green beans, sautéed with water.
- Brine pickles.

- Fried rice using yesterday's rice, with onion, mushrooms, beansprouts and spring onions.
- Sauerkraut.

SUPPER

- Quick miso soup.
- Boiled short-grain rice.
- Aduki beans cooked with kombu, carrot and onion.
- Arame and toasted sesame seeds.
- Pressed salad of lettuce and cucumber with tofu dressing.

- Corn and Chinese cabbage miso soup.
- Pressure-cooked short-grain rice and wheat.
- Waterless-style carrots and kombu.
- Chickpea pâté.
- Cucumber and wakame salad with rice vinegar.
- Strawberry jelly.

BREAKFAST

Wednesday

- Whole oat porridge.
- Brine pickles.

Thursday

- Miso soup from yesterday.

LUNCH

- Rice and wheat from yesterday.
- Steamed carrot and courgette.
- Blanched watercress.

- Sourdough bread.
- Salad of grated carrot and cabbage with tahini dressing.

SUPPER

- Pearl barley and onion miso soup.
- Boiled medium-grain rice.
- Boiled carrot, onion and tofu with kuzu gravy made from the cooking water.
- Blanched spring cabbage cut finely and mixed with sauerkraut.

- Pressure-cooked short-grain rice and barley.
- Lentils cooked with wakame and spring onions.
- Steamed daikon (mouli).
- Blanched salad of cauliflower, celery and watercress with rice vinegar and shoyu dressing.
- Slices of fresh melon.

BREAKFAST

Friday

- Rolled oat porridge.
- Scrambled tofu with spring onions.

Saturday

- Soft millet and onion using yesterday's grain.
- Brine pickles.

LUNCH

- Rice and barley from yesterday.
- Lentils from yesterday.
- Blanched salad from yesterday.

- Corn on the cob.
- Hiziki salad from yesterday.

SUPPER

- Cauliflower and onion miso soup.
- Millet and onion croquettes.
- Sautéed carrot mixed with roasted sesame seeds.
- Hiziki salad with tofu dressing.

- Shoyu broth with carrot matchsticks, onions, mushrooms, tofu, and spring onions.
- Boiled medium-grain rice.
- Shallow-boiled plaice with shoyu, ginger juice and rice vinegar.
- Salad of chopped lettuce, cucumber, radishes and mustard cress with umeboshi dressing.
- Lightly stewed fresh apples with soya-milk custard.

BREAKFAST

Sunday

- Soft rice made from yesterday's grain.
- Blanched salad of cabbage.

LUNCH

- Rice from yesterday mixed with roasted pumpkin seeds.
- Boiled cauliflower, broccoli and runner beans.

SUPPER

- Onion and wakame miso soup.
- Pressure-cooked short-grain rice mixed with blanched peas, green beans and roasted sunflower seeds.
- Waterless-style carrot, turnip and kombu.
- Chickpea salad with onion, celery, radish and lettuce.

WINTER MENUS

BREAKFAST	LUNCH	SUPPER
Monday		
• Soft rice. • Boiled leeks.	• Wholewheat, udon or buckwheat noodles in shoyu broth.	• Daikon and wakame miso soup. • Pressure-cooked short-grain rice. • Aduki beans cooked with kombu and carrots. • Arame and onions. • Pressed salad of finely-cut cabbage with rice vinegar. • Pear and apple crumble.
Tuesday		
• Whole oat porridge. • Steamed watercress.	• Rice from yesterday. • Aduki beans from yesterday. • Blanched salad of cauliflower and Brussels sprouts.	• Lentil soup with onion and parsley. • Millet and onion. • Waterless-style carrot, burdock and kombu. • Boiled kale.

BREAKFAST

Wednesday

- Rolled oat porridge.
- Boiled cabbage.

Thursday

- Soft millet cooked with onion and mushrooms.

LUNCH

- Millet and onion from yesterday.
- Quick sauté of carrot, onion and leek.

- Rice and chestnuts from yesterday.
- Steamed broccoli.

SUPPER

- Shoyu broth with onion, tofu and parsley.
- Pressure-cooked short-grain rice and chestnuts.
- Baked parsnips.
- Hiziki mixed with roasted and sliced almonds.
- Blanched salad of cauliflower, cauliflower greens and spring onions with tofu dressing.
- Oatmeal raisin cookies.

- Aduki bean soup.
- Pressure-cooked short-grain rice and barley.
- Long sauté of carrot, swede and Brussels sprouts.
- Boiled leeks mixed with umeboshi dressing.

BREAKFAST

Friday

- Soft rice made from yesterday's grain cooked with onion and swede.
- Brine pickles.

Saturday

- Miso soup from yesterday with sourdough bread.

LUNCH

- Fried wholewheat spaghetti, udon or buckwheat noodles with onion, leek and tofu.

- Rice from yesterday.
- Boiled carrot, turnip and turnip greens.

SUPPER

- Onion and wakame miso soup.
- Boiled short-grain rice.
- Baked cod with shoyu, mustard and rice vinegar.
- Kombu and carrot rolls.
- Steamed kale and cauliflower cut finely and mixed with sauerkraut.
- Baked apples with soya-milk custard.

- Barley and lentil stew with carrots, onions and Brussels sprouts.
- Blanched salad of Chinese cabbage with rice vinegar and shoyu dressing.

BREAKFAST

Sunday

- Rolled oat porridge.
- Steamed leeks.

LUNCH

- Barley and lentil stew from yesterday.
- Sauerkraut.

SUPPER

- Quick miso soup.
- Pressure-cooked short-grain rice and aduki beans.
- Waterless-style parsnip, swede, Brussels sprouts and kombu.
- Quick sauté of mushrooms, tofu, beansprouts and watercress.

CHAPTER FIFTEEN

RECIPES

The recipes in this chapter can be used in conjunction with the menu plans in chapter 14, or you can use them to plan your own menus. Once you have mastered the recipes in this book, you can increase the variety of your cooking by consulting some of the cookery books listed on page 157.

All the recipes serve 2 to 3 people, except where stated otherwise.

GRAINS

PRESSURE-COOKED BROWN RICE

I cup short- or medium-grain brown rice
1¼-1½ cups water
A pinch of sea salt

Place the rice in a stainless steel pressure-cooker, add water to cover and gently stir with your hand to wash it, then pour off the dirty water. Repeat once or twice, or until the washing water is clear. Add the water and salt, cover, and bring up to pressure. When the pressure is up, turn the heat down very low. A flame deflector can also be placed under the pot, to prevent burning. Cook for 45-50 minutes.

At the end of cooking, turn the heat off and allow the pressure to drop slowly. After 5 minutes the pressure can be allowed to escape by putting a spoon handle under the pressure valve. Take the rice out a spoonful at a time and spread in a serving bowl, carefully separating the individual grains before removing the next spoonful. This rice will have a deliciously sweet nutty flavour.

Variations: Roasted seeds or nuts such as sunflower seeds or almonds can be mixed with the cooked rice. To cook larger amounts, simply increase the quantities so that you still have the same proportion of water and salt to rice.

BOILED RICE

I cup short- or medium-grain brown rice
2 cups water
A pinch of sea salt

Place the rice in a saucepan and wash as for pressure-cooked rice. Add the water and salt, cover with a lid, and bring to the boil. Simmer on very low heat for 50-60 minutes or until all the water has been absorbed. Remove the rice as in the previous recipe.

SOFT RICE

I cup short- or medium-grain brown rice
5 cups water
A pinch of sea salt

Wash the rice and either pressure-cook or boil, as in the above recipes, for 1-1½ hours.

The rice becomes very creamy and makes an excellent breakfast porridge. Soft rice can also be made with cooked rice from the day before by adding 3 cups of water per cup of rice and cooking for 30-45 minutes.

Variations: Soft rice can be cooked with vegetables, such as carrots and onion or Chinese cabbage.

RICE WITH OTHER GRAINS

I cup short- or medium-grain brown rice
¼ cup of pot or pearl barley, or wheat, or millet, or oats
A pinch of sea salt

These combinations can be cooked in the same way as pressure-cooked rice, by placing the grains together in the pot. However, barley, wheat and oats take longer to cook than rice, so they should be soaked for 2-3 hours before adding to the rice.

These make nice variations to plain rice.

RICE WITH BEANS OR DRIED CHESTNUTS

I cup short- or medium-grain brown rice
⅛ cup aduki or black soya beans or dried chestnuts
1¾-2 cups water
2 pinches of sea salt

Spread the beans on a flat plate and pick out any stones or impurities. Place the beans or chestnuts in a pressure-cooker and wash as described above for rice. As beans and dried chestnuts need longer cooking than rice, boil with the water for 30-40 minutes by themselves. Wash the rice separately, then add to the beans or chestnuts with the salt, and pressure-cook for 45-50 minutes. Serve as with plain rice.

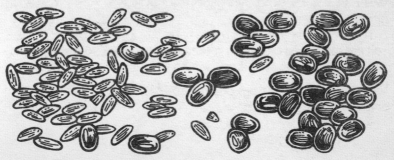

MILLET

I cup millet
2½ cups boiling water
A pinch of sea salt

Wash the millet in the same way as rice, or in a sieve under a tap. Lightly roast in a dry frying pan on a medium heat for 5 minutes until slightly golden. Stir occasionally to prevent burning. Roasting gives millet a beautifully nutty flavour. Add the millet and salt to the boiling water, bring back to the boil, cover and turn the heat to low. Simmer for 30-35 minutes or until all the water has been absorbed. Gently remove a spoonful at a time into a serving bowl.

Variations: Sauté 8 ounces (225g) onions in a little sesame oil until golden and place in the boiling water before the millet. While the millet is still warm it can be shaped in the hands to form burgers or croquettes. Burgers can be fried in a little oil. They are particularly popular with children.

SOFT MILLET

I cup millet
4-5 cups water
A pinch of sea salt

Wash, roast and cook the millet, as in the previous recipe, for 45 minutes or until soft. Soft millet can be used as a breakfast cereal.

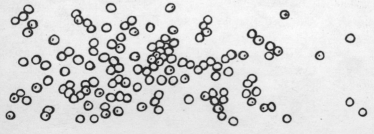

FRIED RICE

2 cups cooked brown rice
1-2 teaspoons sesame oil
1 medium onion, sliced finely
1 medium carrot, sliced finely or cut into matchsticks
4 ounces (100g) mushrooms, sliced finely
1 cup beansprouts
1-2 teaspoons shoyu

Brush a frying pan with the oil and heat for a minute. Spread the onion in the pan, then the other vegetables, and spread the rice on top. Cover the pan and cook on a low flame for 10 minutes. Add the shoyu and cook for another 5 minutes. There should be no need to stir during cooking — just mix together before serving.

Variations: Use other combinations of vegetables. Tofu can also be added to make a complete, balanced meal.

WHOLE OAT PORRIDGE

1 cup whole oats
5-6 cups water
A pinch of sea salt

Wash the oats in the same way as rice and place in a saucepan with the water and salt. Cover and bring to the boil. Reduce the heat to very low and simmer for several hours, or overnight in the winter. Alternatively, cook for 45 minutes the night before, and another 30 minutes in the morning.

This traditional Scottish recipe is extremely creamy and very warming on winter mornings.

ROLLED OAT PORRIDGE

1 cup rolled oats
2½-3 cups water
A pinch of sea salt

It is preferable to use medium rolled or Jumbo oats as they have been milled less, and have a fuller flavour. Place the oats, water and salt in a saucepan, bring to the boil and reduce heat to low. Simmer for 10-30 minutes, depending on the size of the flakes. Garnish with gomasio (sesame salt) or roasted seeds.

Variations: This porridge could occasionally be cooked with sugar-free soya milk for a creamier taste. Barley malt could be added if you want a sweeter taste.

BARLEY AND LENTIL STEW

1 cup barley
3-4 cups water
¼ cup lentils
1 onion, diced
1 cup diced carrots
1 cup chopped Brussels sprouts
3 celery stalks, diced
½ cup button mushrooms
½ teaspoon sea salt

Wash the barley and lentils individually in a sieve under a tap, place all the ingredients in a saucepan, cover and bring to the boil. Reduce heat to low and simmer 1½ hours. For a more warming dish in the winter, once the stew has boiled put it in a casserole with the lid on, and cook in the oven at 250°F (130°C, Gas Mark 1) for 1½-2 hours.

CORN ON THE COB

Steam or boil whole fresh cobs for 10 minutes or until soft. These are delicious as a light grain when they are in season in the summer.

NOODLES AND BROTH

1 packet buckwheat or udon noodles, or wholewheat spaghetti
2 pints (1 litre) water
3-inch (8cm) piece kombu seaweed
3-4 fresh or dried (shitake) mushrooms, sliced
2-3 tablespoons shoyu

Boil 2-3 pints (1-1½ litres) of water, add the noodles and simmer for 10-15 minutes. You can check when they are done by breaking a piece   when the inside and outside are the same colour they are ready. Transfer the noodles from the saucepan into a sieve and rinse under a tap to stop them sticking together.

Start making the broth once the noodles have come to the boil. Wipe the kombu with a damp cloth to remove excess salt and place in a saucepan with the water and mushrooms (dried mushrooms must first be soaked for 15 minutes and their stems removed). Bring to the boil, reduce the heat and simmer for 5 minutes. Remove the kombu, and keep for another recipe. Add the shoyu and simmer 5 minutes more. Place the noodles in the broth to warm up, then serve. Garnish with chopped spring onions, chives or toasted nori seaweed cut into 1-inch (2-3cm) squares.

Variations: Use other vegetables, such as finely sliced carrot and watercress. Small cubes of tofu can also be added.

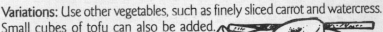

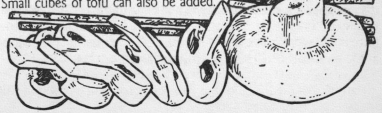

FRIED NOODLES AND VEGETABLES

I packet buckwheat or udon noodles, or wholewheat spaghetti
I tablespoon sesame oil
I medium onion, finely sliced
I cup finely sliced cabbage
½ cup finely sliced mushrooms
½ cup chopped spring onions
I tablespoon shoyu

Cook the noodles as in the previous recipe, rinse and drain. Brush a frying pan with the oil, spread out the onion, cabbage and mushrooms, and the noodles on top. Cover and cook on a low flame for 4-5 minutes. Mix the noodles and vegetables, add the shoyu and cook for 3 minutes. Add spring onions and serve.

Variations: Onion, beansprouts, watercress and tofu.

SOURDOUGH BREAD

3 pounds (1.4kg) wholewheat flour
2 tablespoons sesame oil (optional)
¼ - ½ teaspoon sea salt

Make a starter by mixing ½ cup flour with enough water to make a thin batter. Cover with a damp cloth and stand in a warm place to ferment for 3-4 days or until it smells sour, but not mouldy.

Mix the remaining flour and salt, then rub in the oil. Add the starter and just enough water to form a thick dough, and knead 200-300 times. Oil 2 bread pans with sesame oil and put the dough in them. Cover with a damp cloth and leave to sit in a warm place for 8-12 hours or until it has risen to twice the size. Bake at 300°F (150°C, Gas Mark 3) for 15 minutes and then at 350°F (180°C, Gas Mark 4) for 1¼-1½ hours.

Sourdough bread can be very sweet and delicious. If you are making it regularly, remove a little of the kneaded dough and mix with a little water to begin your next starter.

SOUPS

VEGETABLE MISO SOUP

½ cup onions thinly sliced
3-4-inch (8-10cm) piece of wakame seaweed
1 pint (550ml) water
½-1 tablespoon miso

Quickly rinse the wakame in water to remove excess salt, and soak in ½ cup water for 5 minutes, then slice into ½-inch (1cm) pieces. Place the wakame with its soaking water and onions in a saucepan and add the rest of the water. Bring to the boil, cover, and simmer for 10-15 minutes or until tender. Reduce flame to very low so there is no bubbling. Purée the miso with ¼ cup of the soup and return to the soup. Allow to cook for 3-4 minutes without bubbling to preserve the beneficial enzymes in the miso, and serve. Garnish with chopped parsley, spring onions or watercress, or grated root ginger.

The soup should not taste too salty nor too bland. A little more miso will be needed in the winter, and a little less in the summer. Barley miso is the most balanced and the best to use regularly, hatcho (100% soya bean) and brown rice can be used occasionally. Hatcho miso is more yang and can be used more often in the winter; brown rice miso is more yin and can be used more often in the summer.

Variations: cauliflower and onion; wakame and daikon (mouli); corn cut from a cob and Chinese cabbage.

QUICK MISO SOUP

⅓ cup chopped spring onions
1 pint (550ml) water
1 sheet of nori seaweed cut into 1-inch (2-3cm) squares
½-1 tablespoon miso

Boil the water, reduce the flame to very low so there is no bubbling. Remove ¼ cup and purée the miso in it, then return to the pan. Add the spring onions and cook for 3-4 minutes. Add nori and serve.

SHOYU BROTH

3-inch (8cm) piece of kombu seaweed
3-4 fresh or dried (shitake) mushrooms, sliced
½ cup cubed tofu
¼ cup chopped spring onions
1 pint (550ml) water
1-2 tablespoons shoyu

If you are using dried mushrooms, soak them for 10 minutes and cut off the stalks. Wipe the kombu with a damp cloth to remove excess salt and place with the water in a pot. Simmer for 5 minutes (this adds minerals and much flavour). Remove the kombu and use in another recipe. Add the mushrooms and tofu, simmer for 5-10 minutes. Add the shoyu, and simmer for 2-3 minutes more. Add the spring onions and serve.

Variations: Onion, tofu and watercress; Chinese cabbage and chives; sautéed onion and parsley.

ADUKI BEAN SOUP

1 cup aduki beans
2-inch (5cm) piece of kombu seaweed
2 medium onions, sliced
2 medium carrots, sliced
2 pints (1 litre) water
½-1 tablespoon shoyu

Wipe the excess salt off the kombu with a damp cloth, soak for 10-15 minutes and slice into thin strips. Put the beans on a flat plate, pick out stones and impurities, then wash in a sieve under a tap. Put the kombu, beans and water in a saucepan, bring to the boil, cover and reduce the heat to low. Simmer for 1 hour. Add the onion, carrot and shoyu and simmer for 30 minutes more. Garnish with chopped spring onions or parsley, and serve.

Variations: Vary the vegetables, using parsnip and leek, or carrot and celery, for example.

LENTIL SOUP

1 cup green or brown lentils
2 medium onions, diced
1 carrot, diced
¼ cup chopped parsley
2 pints (1 litre) water
A pinch of sea salt
½-1 tablespoon shoyu

Put the lentils on a flat plate, pick out stones and impurities then wash the lentils in a sieve under a tap. Spread the onion on the bottom of a saucepan, then add the carrot, and the lentils on top. Add the water and a pinch of salt and bring to the boil. Reduce flame to low, cover and simmer for 50 minutes. Add the parsley and shoyu, simmer for 10 minutes more and serve.

Variations: The same recipe can be used to make a creamy split pea soup, using 1 cup split peas in place of the lentils.

PEARL BARLEY AND ONION SOUP

½ cup pearl barley
3 medium onions, sliced thinly
1 teaspoon sesame oil
2 pints (1 litre) water
A pinch of sea salt
1-2 tablespoons shoyu

Wash the barley, then boil in the water for 45 minutes. Sauté the onions in the oil with a pinch of salt until golden brown. Add the onions to the barley and cook for another 20 minutes. Add the shoyu and cook for 10 minutes more. Garnish with chopped parsley or nori seaweed cut into 1-inch (2-3cm) squares.

VEGETABLES

BOILING

Put 1-2 inches (2-5cm) of water in a saucepan, add a pinch of salt (optional) and bring to the boil. Add the vegetables for between 1 and 10 minutes, then remove and serve. Keep the remaining water for a soup or other recipe.

Most vegetables can be cooked in this way. Some cook very fast — for example, watercress and spring onions — and need only 1-2 minutes. Others, like carrots and swede, need longer.

Tasty combinations of boiled vegetables include broccoli and cauliflower; carrots, onions and peas; cabbage, corn and tofu; leeks with umeboshi (pickled plums).

STEAMING

Put ½-inch (1cm) of water in a saucepan and then a vegetable steamer. Add sliced vegetables and sprinkle with a pinch of sea salt (optional). Cover, bring to the boil, and steam for 2-7 minutes. Remove the vegetables and serve. Save the remaining water for other dishes.

Green vegetables generally take 1-4 minutes steaming, round and root vegetables take a little longer. If you do not have a steamer, put ½ inch (1cm) of water in a pot, add the vegetables and salt, cover and steam.

This is an ideal way of cooking greens like kale, spring cabbage, Chinese cabbage, watercress, and turnip tops, and can be used frequently.

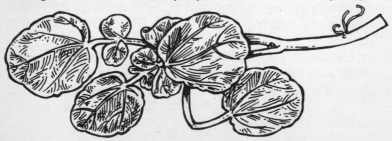

BAKING

8 ounces (225g) carrots, parsnips or Hokkaido pumpkin, cut in thick slices
1-2 teaspoons shoyu

Place the vegetables on a baking tray, add ¼-½ inch (½-1cm) of water and sprinkle the shoyu over the vegetables. Bake at 400°F (200°C, Gas Mark 6) for 40 minutes or until soft. Add more water if necessary.

These vegetables become very sweet cooked in this way.

QUICK SAUTÉ

½ cup carrot, cut in thin matchsticks
½ cup thinly sliced onions
½ cup thinly sliced cabbage
½ cup beansprouts
¼ cup thinly sliced mushrooms
1-2 teaspoons sesame oil
1-2 pinches of sea salt
1-2 teaspoons shoyu
1-2 teaspoons rice vinegar

Brush a frying pan with the oil and heat for 1 minute. Add the vegetables and sprinkle the salt over them. Cook for 5 minutes on a medium flame, gently turning the vegetables occasionally. Add the shoyu and vinegar and cook for 1-2 minutes more, then serve. The vegetables should be tender, but still crisp.

If you are limiting the amount of oil that you eat, replace the oil with 2-3 tablespoons of water.

Variations: Onion, Chinese cabbage, corn, watercress and tofu; parsnip, onion, celery and broccoli.

LONG SAUTÉ

½ cup carrot, cut in thick matchsticks or in slices
½ cup broccoli, cut into pieces
½ cup onion, cut in thick slices
½ cup cauliflower, cut into pieces
1-2 teaspoons sesame oil
1-2 pinches of sea salt
1-2 teaspoons shoyu

Brush a pan with the oil and heat for 1 minute. Add the vegetables, sprinkle the salt over them, and cook on a medium heat for 5 minutes, turning occasionally. Add water to just cover the bottom of the pan. Cover and cook for 10-15 minutes, adding more water if necessary to prevent burning. Add shoyu and cook for 2-3 minutes more without a cover to allow any remaining water to evaporate.

Variations: Parsnip, onion, cabbage and tofu; burdock and carrot; carrot and roasted sesame seeds.

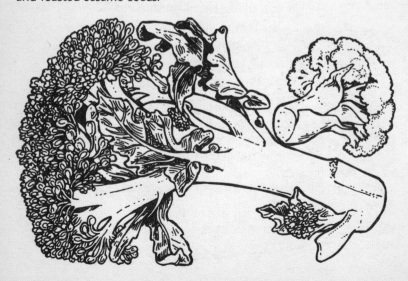

WATERLESS STYLE

6-inch (15cm) piece of kombu seaweed
1 carrot, cut in 1-2 inch (2-5cm) chunks
1 medium onion, cut in quarters
¼ cabbage, cut in 1-2 inch (2-5cm) wide slices through the stem
A pinch of sea salt
1-2 teaspoons shoyu

Wipe the kombu with a damp cloth to remove excess salt, soak for 10-20 minutes and cut into 1-inch (2-3cm) pieces. Put the kombu in the bottom of a heavy pot that has a tight fitting lid. Add the vegetables, ½ inch (1cm) of water, and salt. Cover and bring to the boil, then turn to medium low heat and cook for 15-30 minutes. If necessary, add more water to prevent burning. Add shoyu and cook for 3 minutes longer. Any juice left can be served with the vegetables, and is very delicious.

This method of cooking with little water is more yang, and is very strengthening.

Variations: Parsnip, onion and cabbage; burdock, swede and cauliflower.

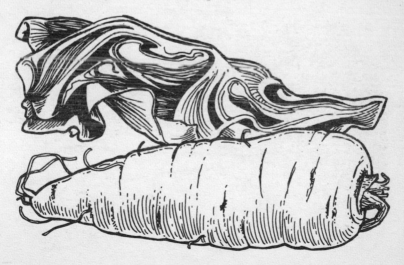

BLANCHED SALAD

I cup sliced Chinese cabbage
½ cup sliced onion
½ cup thinly sliced carrot
½ cup sliced celery
I bunch watercress
I-2 pinches of sea salt

Put 1-2 inches (2-5cm) of water in a saucepan, add the salt and bring to the boil. Blanch the vegetables one at a time, starting with the mildest tasting, so that each will keep its distinctive flavour. Start by putting the Chinese cabbage in, boil for I minute, and remove with a wire mesh scoop or slotted spoon. Next blanch the onion, then the carrot, followed by the celery. Lastly do the watercress for a few seconds only. As you remove each vegetable, spread it out on a dish to cool so that it retains its bright colour.

Mix the vegetables together and add a dressing such as rice vinegar and shoyu or tofu dressing.

Variations: Most vegetables can be prepared in this way; for example, green beans, onion and fresh peas, or cauliflower and broccoli.

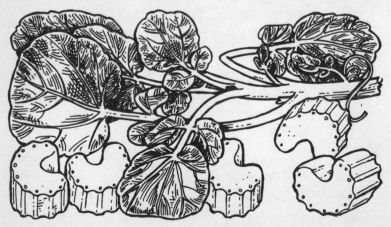

PRESSED SALAD

½ lettuce, shredded
½ cucumber, thinly sliced
½ cup thinly sliced radishes
2 pinches of sea salt

Mix the cut vegetables and salt together. They can be pressed in one of three ways: firstly, in a commercial salad press; secondly, by placing a saucer on the vegetables with a stone or heavy jar on top; and thirdly, by repeatedly pressing on them with the palm of your hand. The first two methods take 2-3 hours, the third about 5 minutes. After pressing, squeeze the excess water from the vegetables, and add rice vinegar or a dressing

Variations: Red radish and cucumber; lettuce, celery and daikon (mouli).

BRINE PICKLES

½ cup carrots
2 medium onions
1 cup cauliflower florets
1 cup sliced white cabbage
1 pint (550ml) water
2 teaspoons sea salt

To make the brine, boil the salt in the water until it dissolves, then allow to cool. Slice the vegetables thinly and pack tightly in a glass or ceramic jar. Add brine to cover the vegetables and put a stone or cup on top to keep them under the surface.

Store in a warm place for 5-10 days, tasting a piece occasionally. When the raw taste is replaced by a sharp, slightly sour taste they are done. Store in a refrigerator or cool place, and enjoy them over the next 2 or 3 weeks.

Variations: Onion, celery and green beans; pickling onions.

BEANS

ADUKI BEANS

I cup aduki beans
4-inch (10cm) piece of kombu seaweed
4 cups of water
¼ - ½ teaspoon sea salt or 1-2 teaspoons shoyu

Spread the beans on a flat plate and pick out stones and impurities. Wash in a sieve under the tap. Wipe the kombu with a damp cloth and place it in the bottom of a saucepan. Add the beans and water and cover. Bring to the boil, turn the heat to low, and simmer for I hour. Add more water if needed, to keep the beans covered. Add the salt or shoyu and cook for 20-30 minutes more. Remove the cover and simmer until all the liquid has gone.

Variations: Just before adding the salt or shoyu, add chunks of carrot and onion, or Hokkaido pumpkin.

SCRAMBLED TOFU

I cake of tofu
I teaspoon sesame oil
¼ - ½ cup chopped spring onions or parsley
½-1 teaspoon shoyu

Brush a frying pan with the oil and heat for I minute. Add the tofu, breaking it up with a wooden spoon. Cook on a medium heat for 3-4 minutes, turning occasionally. Add the shoyu and spring onions and cook for I minute more, then serve.

CHICKPEAS

I cup chickpeas
4-inch (10cm) piece of wakame seaweed
3 cups water
¼-½ teaspoon sea salt or 1-2 teaspoons shoyu

Chickpeas are usually pressure-cooked to speed up the long cooking time they require. Spread them on a flat plate and pick out the impurities, then wash in a sieve under the tap and soak for 12 hours.

Wipe the wakame with a damp cloth and place in a pressure-cooker, followed by the chickpeas and water. Cover, bring to pressure, turn the heat to low and cook for 1½ hours.

Remove the pressure-cooker from the heat and cool by running cold water over it. Remove the cover, add salt or shoyu, and simmer for 30-40 minutes, by which time all the liquid should have gone.

Variations: Just before adding the salt or shoyu, add diced carrot and onion, or Hokkaido pumpkin. Chopped parsley or spring onions can also be added at the end of cooking.

CHICKPEA SALAD

I cup of chickpeas, cooked as above
½ cup sliced celery
½ cup sliced onion
½ cup sliced radishes
I cup shredded lettuce
2 tablespoons tahini
2 tablespoons rice vinegar
I teaspoon mustard, freshly ground seeds or powder
2 teaspoons shoyu

Mix the chickpeas and vegetables together. Purée the tahini by slowly adding the vinegar and shoyu, stir in the mustard, and mix into the salad.

CHICKPEA PÂTÉ

I cup chickpeas, cooked as above
I tablespoon tahini
I teaspoon mustard, freshly ground seeds or powder
I tablespoon rice vinegar
I teaspoon shoyu
¼ cup chopped chives or parsley

Purée all the ingredients together in a suribachi (Japanese mortar) or in a blender. Serve with the chives or parsley as a garnish.

LENTILS

I cup green or brown lentils
3-inch (8cm) piece of wakame seaweed
2½-3 cups water
¼ cup chopped parsley or spring onions
¼ teaspoon sea salt or I-2 teaspoons shoyu

Spread the lentils on a flat plate and pick out stones and impurities, then wash in a sieve under the tap. Wipe the wakame with a damp cloth to remove excess salt, place in a saucepan, add the lentils and then the water. Cover and bring to the boil. Turn the heat to low and simmer for 30 minutes. Add the salt or shoyu and cook for 20-30 minutes more. Remove the cover and allow any remaining liquid to cook off. Add parsley or spring onions and serve.

Variations: Diced vegetables can be added just before adding the salt or shoyu; for example, carrot and onion or onion and celery.

SEA VEGETABLES

CUCUMBER AND WAKAME SALAD

½ cucumber
2 pinches of sea salt
10 inches (25cm) of wakame seaweed
2 teaspoons rice vinegar

Wash the cucumber and slice finely. Place in a bowl, add water to just cover and sprinkle on the salt. Leave for 30-45 minutes. Quickly wash the wakame to remove excess salt, soak for 10 minutes, then cut into 1-inch (2-3cm) pieces. Keep the wakame soaking water for a soup or other dish, as it will contain many minerals. Drain the cucumber and mix with the wakame. Add the rice vinegar and serve.

Variations: Soaked wakame can be included in the ingredients of any pressed or raw salad to add a quite different colour and taste.

ARAME

½ cup dried arame
1 medium onion, sliced
1 medium carrot, sliced or cut in matchsticks
1-2 teaspoons shoyu

Quickly wash the arame in water to remove excess salt. Place in a bowl, cover with water and soak for 10 minutes. Remove the arame and slice into 1-2 inch (2-5cm) pieces. Place the onion and carrot in a saucepan, and the arame on top. Add the soaking water and enough additional water to just cover the arame. Cover, bring to the boil, reduce the heat to low and simmer for 30 minutes. Add the shoyu and simmer without a lid until all the water has gone. Mix together only at the end, and serve.

Variations: Burdock and onion or salsify and onion; carrot and roasted sesame seeds or roasted and sliced almonds.

HIZIKI

Cook as for arame, but with a longer total cooking time of 50-60 minutes. Hiziki is also excellent when combined with vegetables or roasted seeds or nuts.

HIZIKI SALAD

½ cup dried hiziki
½ cup thinly sliced onion
½ cup thinly sliced cauliflower
½ cup thinly sliced celery
¼ cup roasted sunflower seeds

Cook the hiziki as above, without any vegetables. Blanch the vegetables as described in the Blanched Salad recipe. Mix the hiziki, vegetables and seeds together and serve. A dressing such as tofu dressing could be added if desired.

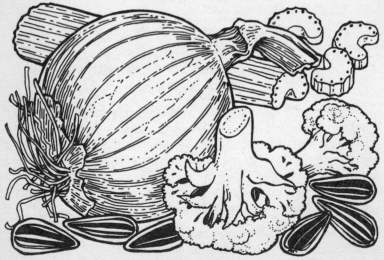

KOMBU AND CARROT ROLLS

2 large carrots, cut into 2-inch (5cm) pieces
4-inch (10cm) strip of dried kombu per piece of carrot
6-inch (15cm) piece of wakame stem or gourd strip per
piece of carrot
1-2 teaspoons shoyu

Wipe the kombu with a damp cloth to remove excess salt and soak for 10 minutes or until soft. Roll each piece of carrot in a piece of kombu and tie in the centre with the wakame stem or gourd strip. Arrange all the rolls on the bottom of a saucepan and half cover with water. Cover, bring to the boil, turn the heat to medium low and simmer for 20-30 minutes. Add the shoyu and cook for 10 minutes more without a lid so that all the water is cooked away.

Variations: You can also try making rolls with parsnips, burdock, salsify or daikon (mouli).

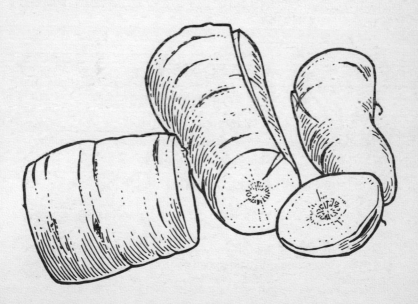

FISH

POACHED FISH

I plaice fillet
1-2 tablespoons shoyu
I teaspoon ginger juice squeezed from grated root ginger
I tablespoon rice vinegar

Wash the fish and marinate in the shoyu, vinegar and ginger juice for I hour. Put the fish in a frying pan, add the marinade and enough water to half cover the fish. Simmer on a medium flame for 2-3 minutes, turn over and simmer for another 2-3 minutes or until the fish is cooked all the way through. Serve with a salad or plenty of lightly cooked greens.

If you have less time, instead of marinating the fish you can just add the shoyu, vinegar and ginger juice when it is cooking.

Variations: The same method can be used to cook cod, haddock, flounder, trout and other white fish.

BAKED FISH

I cod fillet
1-2 tablespoons shoyu
¼ teaspoon freshly ground mustard seeds or mustard powder
I tablespoon rice vinegar

Wash and marinate the fish as above. Place on a baking tray, add the marinade and enough water to half cover the fish. Bake in an oven at 400°F (200°C, Gas Mark 6) for 10-20 minutes or until the fish is cooked through.

Instead of marinating the fish you can also bake it straight away, with the shoyu, vinegar and mustard added to it in the baking tray.

Variations: Any white fish can be cooked using this method.

SAUCES AND DRESSINGS

KUZU GRAVY

2 cups of vegetable cooking water or plain water
¼ cup thinly sliced mushrooms
1 tablespoon kuzu
1-2 teaspoons shoyu

Heat the water in a frying pan, add the mushrooms and shoyu and simmer for 5 minutes. Purée the kuzu in 3 tablespoons of cold water. Remove the pan from the heat and stir in the kuzu. Return the pan to the heat and simmer for 5 minutes, gently stirring to prevent lumps forming. Serve over vegetables, noodles, and other dishes.

Variations: For a different taste, add sautéed onions or a little ginger juice squeezed from grated root ginger.

TOFU DRESSING

1 cake tofu
¼ onion, diced finely
½-1 teaspoon miso
1-2 teaspoons rice vinegar
¼ cup chopped spring onions, parsley or chives

Purée the miso in 1-2 tablespoons water with a suribashi (Japanese mortar) or blender. Add the onion and purée it with the miso. Add the tofu and rice vinegar and purée until creamy, adding a little water if necessary. Mix in the spring onions, parsley or chives. Serve on blanched, pressed or raw salads.

VINEGAR AND SHOYU DRESSING

3 teaspoons rice vinegar
1 teaspoon shoyu

Mix the vinegar and shoyu together, and serve over salads or steamed vegetables.

TAHINI DRESSING

2 tablespoons tahini
1 tablespoon shoyu
¼ onion diced finely

Purée the onion, tahini and shoyu in a pestle and mortar or suribashi. Slowly mix in enough water to make a thin paste. Serve on blanched, pressed or raw salads.

UMEBOSHI (PICKLED PLUM) DRESSING

2 umeboshi or 2 teaspoons umeboshi paste

Purée the flesh of the plums or the paste with a few teaspoons of water until a thin, smooth paste is obtained. Use on salads and vegetable dishes.

CONDIMENTS

GOMASIO (SESAME SALT)

1 teaspoon fine sea salt
10-14 teaspoons sesame seeds

Roast the salt in a frying pan on a medium heat for 5 minutes, then put into a mortar or suribashi. Roast the sesame seeds in the pan until they become lightly golden and can be easily crushed between two fingers. Stir frequently to get even roasting. If the seeds begin to pop, turn the heat lower. Put the seeds in the mortar or suribashi and grind with the salt until about two-thirds of the seeds have been crushed.

Home-made gomasio has a delicious nutty fragrance and taste, and can be sprinkled on grains, breakfast porridge, noodles and vegetable dishes. If it is stored in an airtight jar it will stay fresh for 1-2 weeks. You may well want to make up 2 or 3 times the quantities given above.

ROASTED SEEDS AND NUTS

Seeds such as sesame, sunflower and pumpkin are most easily roasted in a dry frying pan. Nuts like almonds, walnuts, hazels and peanuts may be roasted in a pan, or in an oven which makes even roasting easier.

When roasting in a pan, cook on a medium low heat for 5-10 minutes, stirring frequently to obtain even roasting. When done, seeds or nuts are slightly darker in colour, and have a fragrant aroma and taste. A few drops of shoyu can be added a minute before the end of cooking for seasoning.

When roasting in the oven, put the nuts on a baking tray and bake for 5-10 minutes at 400°F (200°C, Gas Mark 6), or until they become slightly darker in colour with a fragrant aroma.

Seeds and nuts can be used as snacks, in desserts, or in grain and vegetable dishes.

DESSERTS

FRUIT JELLY (KANTEN)

3 sweet apples, sliced
2 cups water
3 tablespoons concentrated apple juice
1 pinch sea salt
Agar-agar flakes or powder

Wash and slice the apples, place in a saucepan with the water, juice and salt. Add the amount of agar-agar indicated by directions on the packet (it varies from make to make). Bring to a boil while stirring, reduce heat to low and simmer 5-10 minutes. Rinse a mould with cold water and pour in the fruit. Place in a refrigerator or cool place to harden, then turn out on a flat serving dish.

Variations: Any fresh or dried fruits can be put in this jelly, such as pears, peaches or dried apricots. Dried fruits will need to be cooked 5-10 minutes longer to soften.

BAKED APPLES

Sweet apples
1 tablespoon sultanas per apple
1 teaspoon tahini per apple
1 teaspoon barley malt (malt extract) per apple
A pinch of sea salt per apple

Core the apples from one end only. Mix the sultanas, tahini, malt and salt together in a bowl and fill the apples. Place on a baking tray and bake in the oven at 375°F (190°C, Gas Mark 5) for 15 minutes or until soft.

SOYA MILK CUSTARD

1½ cups sugar-free soya milk
1 tablespoon concentrated apple juice
1 tablespoon kuzu
5-6 drops vanilla essence (optional)

Put the soya milk, apple juice and vanilla in a saucepan and bring to the boil. Remove from the heat. Purée the kuzu in 2-3 tablespoons cold water and add to the saucepan. Return the pan to a low heat and simmer for 5 minutes, stirring constantly to prevent lumps forming.

More or less kuzu can be added, depending on how thick you like your custard! It is delicious on baked apples, pear and apple crumble, or just on its own.

STEWED FRUIT

1 lb (450g) fresh sweet apples or 4 oz (100g) dried apples, pears, apricots or other fruit
1 tablespoon barley malt (malt extract)
A pinch of sea salt
1 tablespoon kuzu (optional)

If you are using fresh apples, remove the cores and slice thinly. Boil in ½ cup water with the salt and malt for 5 minutes. If there is some liquid left, purée the kuzu in 2-3 tablespoons cold water and add to the apple. Stir constantly until it has thickened, and serve.

If you are using dried fruit, soak it in a bowl with enough water to cover the fruit for 20-30 minutes, then put the fruit, soaking water and salt into a saucepan and simmer until soft. Add the malt 2 minutes before the end of cooking. If there is some liquid left, add the kuzu as described above, and serve.

RICE PUDDING

2 cups cooked short- or medium-grain rice
¼ cup sultanas
3 tablespoons barley malt (malt extract)
A pinch of sea salt
4 cups water

Place all the ingredients in a saucepan and simmer for 30 minutes. Pour into a baking dish and bake at 325°F (170°C, Gas Mark 3) for 30-40 minutes. Serve with chopped roasted nuts on top.

PEAR AND APPLE CRUMBLE

2 sweet apples, sliced
2 pears, sliced
3 tablespoons barley malt (malt extract)
I teaspoon kuzu
3 cups rolled oats
3 tablespoons sesame oil
¼ teaspoon sea salt

Put the fruit with ½ cup of water in a saucepan and bring to the boil. Remove from the heat. Purée the kuzu in 2-3 tablespoons cold water and add to the saucepan. Replace the pan on a low heat, simmer for 3-4 minutes, stirring constantly to prevent lumps forming. Pour into a baking dish.

To prepare the crumble, mix the rolled oats and salt, then rub in the oil. Warm the malt and mix with the oats. Spread over the fruit. Bake in the oven at 350°F (180°C, Gas Mark 4) for 30-45 minutes.

Variations: Many fruits can be cooked in a crumble; for example, apple and blackberries, dried peaches and apricots.

OATMEAL RAISIN COOKIES

2 cups rolled oats
½ cup wholemeal flour
2 tablespoons sesame oil
2 tablespoons barley malt (malt extract)
¼ cup raisins
¼ teaspoon sea salt

Simmer the raisins, with just enough water to cover them, for 5 minutes. Mix the rolled oats, flour and salt, then rub in the oil. Add the raisins with the cooking liquid and malt, and stir together. Add enough water to make a thick batter. Lightly brush a baking tray with oil and form cookies about ¼ inch (½ cm) thick on it. Bake at 375°F (190°C, Gas Mark 5) for 25 minutes or until golden brown.

Variations: You can use this basic recipe to make many different kinds of cookies; for example, walnut and raisin, apple and ginger, or hazelnut and sultana.

TEA

THREE-YEAR TWIG TEA (Bancha or Kukicha)

Simmer 1-2 tablespoons of tea with 2 pints (1 litre) of water for 5 minutes. Pour into a cup through a tea strainer. Return the twigs to the pot, add more water and a few more twigs for your next brew. Experiment with the strength that you prefer — some people like this tea weak while others prefer it strong.

APPENDIX

FURTHER READING

General Reading

Aihara, Herman. *Acid and Alkaline*, Oroville, CA; George Ohsawa Macrobiotic Foundation, 1980.

_____. *Basic Macrobiotics*, Tokyo; Japan Publications Inc., 1985.

Fukuoka, Masanobu. *The One-Straw Revolution*. Emmaus, PA; Rodale Press, 1978.

_____. *The Natural Way Of Farming*. Tokyo; Japan Publications Inc., 1985.

Heidenry, Carolyn, *An Introduction To Macrobiotics*. Boston; Aladdin Press, 1984.

_____. *Making The Transition To A Macrobiotic Diet*. Boston; Aladdin Press, 1985.

Kushi, Aveline, and Michio Kushi. *Macrobiotic Child Care and Family Health*. Tokyo; Japan Publications Inc., 1985.

_____. *Macrobiotic Pregnancy and Care of the Newborn Child*. Tokyo; Japan Publications Inc., 1984.

Kushi, Michio. *The Book of Do-in: Exercise for Physical and Spiritual Development*. Tokyo; Japan Publications Inc., 1979.

_____. *The Book of Macrobiotics*. Tokyo; Japan Publications Inc., 1977.

_____. *Michio Kushi On The Greater View: Collected Thoughts and Ideas on Macrobiotics and Humanity*. Wayne, NJ.; Avery Publishing Group Inc. 1986.

_____. *Your Face Never Lies: An Introduction to Oriental Diagnosis*. Wayne, NJ.; Avery Publishing Group Inc., 1983.

_____, with Alex Jack. *The Cancer Prevention Diet*. Wellingborough, Thorsons Publishing Group, 1984.

Miller, Saul. *Food for Thought: A New Look at Food & Behaviour*. NJ.; Prentice-Hall Inc., 1985.

Tara, William. *Macrobiotics and Human Behaviour*. Tokyo, Japan Publications Inc., 1985.

Cookery Books

Cowmeadow, Michele. *Macrobiotic Cooking*. Penzance; Cornish Connection, 1985.

_____. *Macrobiotic Desserts*. Penzance; Cornish Connection, 1986.

Esko, Wendy. *Introducing Macrobiotic Cooking*. Tokyo; Japan Publications Inc., 1978.

Kushi, Aveline. *Aveline Kushi's Complete Guide to Macrobiotic Cooking*. New York; Warner Books, 1985.

Bradford, Peter and Montse. *Cooking With Sea Vegetables*. Wellingborough; Thorsons Publishing Group, 1985.

Periodicals

East West Journal. Brookline, Massachusetts, USA.

Macromuse. 11119 Rockville Park, Suite 321, Rockville, MD 20852, USA.

Scientific Reports

Dietary Goals for the United States. Washington, DC.; Select Committee on Nutrition and Human Needs, US Senate. Government Printing Office, 1977.

Proposals for Nutritional Guidelines for Health Education in Britain. London; NACNE, 1983.

These books can all be obtained from the following shops by mail order, or from your local bookshop.

In the UK:
Genesis Books
188 Old Street
London EC1V 9BP
Tel: 01-250-1868

In the USA:
Redwing Book Company
44 Linden Street
Brookline, Ma 02146
Tel: 617-738-4664

INFORMATION ON CLASSES AND MACROBIOTIC COUNSELLORS

In the UK:
The Kushi Institute
188 Old Street
London EC1V 9BP
Tel: 01-251-4076

In the USA:
Macrobiotics International
17 Station Street
Brookline, MA 02147
Tel: 617-738-0045

MAIL ORDER SUPPLIES

If you have problems obtaining any of the foods mentioned in this book, they can be obtained by mail order from the companies below. They also supply foods wholesale, so you may be able to get your local health or whole food shop to buy them.

UK Supplier
Clearspring Natural Grocery
196 Old Street
London EC1V 9BP
Tel: 01-250-1708

USA Supplier
Mountain Ark Trading Company
120 South East Street
Fayetteville, AR 72701.
Tel: 501-442-7191

INDEX